"One Picture is worth a thousand words"

Albert Einstein

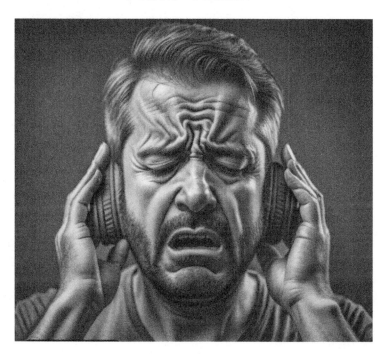

Tackling Tinnitus

By Jake Sutton

Introduction

With a world full of problems, famine, disease, natural disaster, war zones, homelessness and poverty to name but a few, when you try to explain to somebody that you suffer with tinnitus you are unlikely to receive a great deal of sympathy - if any at all. Usually, those who do find it within themselves to sympathise are those who have sufferer or continue to suffer with tinnitus. I'd like to reassure you at a very early stage in this book that I am one of those who sit on the side of sympathy. You may well know just like me that regardless of my sympathetic stance this doesn't solve tinnitus on its own, although hopefully by reading this book I can help you to take some huge strides towards solving that problem. Before you read on you should know I am not a doctor or any kind of medical practitioner but since neither doctors nor medical practitioners seem to know a hard and fast cure for tinnitus, I guess I don't need to be fully medically certified to talk about my experiences, research and solutions. In fact, as a former severe tinnitus sufferer I feel perhaps more qualified to help you, but like most things in life the proof will certainly be in the pudding.

Let me begin by explaining and expanding on my own my tinnitus experiences. My symptoms began when I was 31 years old, I can remember the day, the place and even what I was doing. It was a weekend morning and with two very young children in my house I'd woken to the usual screams, laughter and breakfast time chaos. The house wasn't in silence, it never really is on any day of the week but on this particular morning there was a buzz echoing through my ears which appeared to come completely out of nowhere. At first was hard to distinguish above all of the other general house hold noises, but unmistakeably there was a definite buzz/ringing that just wouldn't seem to go away. At that time in my life, I didn't really have anything to compare it too but perhaps the best way to describe it would be similar to the noise you get in your ears following a night of heavy music and alcohol, the type of noise that would disappear after a few hours or even a day, wouldn't it? Back in my late teens and throughout my twenties, before children, marriage and responsibility was my priority I would sometimes wake to something similar, a ringing in both ears from the deafening music the night before or even perhaps a crazy loud family party but nothing was ever permanent, the ringing in my ears would last a day, maybe two days maximum but then it would ordinarily stop. I had experienced this type of thing on a few occasions and I do wonder those nights out played had an impact in later life. On this occasion though certainly not having been to a party or a nightclub or any parties, there really wasn't any obvious explanation. I can vividly remember brushing it off and the ringing disappearing into the general noise of the day. As the dishes were put away, the kids put to bed

4

and the tv switched off the house begun to fall silent and almost immediately there it was waiting for me, my nemesis for the next 5 years - tinnitus, it had patiently waited for silence to descend upon my home. I lay in bed that night with nothing but pure ringing in my ears, as frustrating as this was, I still felt that these recognisable symptoms would only be temporary, I naively thought 'surely a good night's sleep and I would wake up and forget all about it'. The more I tried to ignore it, the harder and louder it would manifest. Sadly, little could prepare me for battle and anguish that would lay ahead of me in the next few years. As I woke the next day, there it was lingering in the background, an un-mistakable fuzz, buzz, ringing that just wouldn't go away, this isn't normal I thought, isn't it? I began to search my mind for obvious explanations. Am I overly stressed? too much caffeine maybe? I wasn't overly stressed and I hadn't consumed more than my two or three cups of coffee which was nothing more or less than usual. As the days passed the ringing, buzzing remained hard and fast 24/7. To appease my own sanity, I started to introduce the process of elimination, for my own sanity I needed to know why on earth this was happening to me. One-by-one, day-by-day I begun eliminating probable causes. I began by cutting out the tea and coffee, making a conscious effort to avoid getting unnecessarily stressed, re-assed my work load, monitored sleep patterns. Weeks begun to pass but sadly the early self-sacrifices didn't appear to make any tangible difference. Maybe I needed to introduce some positive lifestyle changes to repair the damage? I started introducing calming nature walks, made amendments to my diet by introducing a lorry load more fruit vegetables, joined the local gym and took up yoga. Whatever I tried it never seemed to help. After the initial token gesture lifestyle amendments then came the many doctors' appointments and various professional consultations. After five or six visits to the GP I was eventually referred to the ENT (Ear Nose & Throat) department at my local hospital. Once referred and professionally assessed not long after I was officially diagnosed with a severe case of tinnitus. In the early stages of my diagnoses, I held genuine hope that I wouldn't need to worry much as whatever I couldn't solve with lifestyle changes could be solved with medication or some other medical intervention, how wrong I was. I cannot express the sadness, anguish and upset I felt when I was told by the GP and the ENT that no immediate cure existed for tinnitus. I have to admit that initially I refused to accept the diagnoses and entered a period of denial. Naturally by failing to accept what I had been told my own research commenced and I became quicky frustrated to find that the opinion was shared by various specialists globally was unanimous - no proven definitive cures existed. All research led to the same place (mainly on google – more on that in a moment) there appeared to be a real lack of hope, advice or help available no matter where I looked. The ENT department offered me counselling which I half-heartedly accepted in the belief it would have no impact but after some reluctant participation I didn't find it to be of help to me. I was totally broken, there was no escape from this relentless buzzing which despite trying to ignore it had begun to severely impact upon my life, there had to be another way to deal with this surely? I think most ailments in life allow at least some escape as you can take pain relief, surgery or utilise distraction but with tinnitus it's so hard to deal with as it's inside your head meaning no escape, it's incredibly frustrating and I genuinely begun to understand how some of the more extreme cases of Tinnitus have been known to drive people to suicide. As the days turned into weeks, the weeks into months, and eventually the months into years, the frustration turned to despair. It is safe to say in the few years that followed I ticked off everything in my immediate power to rid myself of the ringing in my ears. I even pushed for a CT scan via the hospital neurology department which I was eventually granted. If you have tried to get a CT referral, you'll know just how difficult this can be, especially as CT scans are not offered as standard especially not for matters related to tinnitus, eventually though my persistence paid off. I was referred to the neurology department at the hospital which led to a scan and full diagnostic review of my symptoms. Even though I felt that a CT wouldn't give me any definitive solutions for my own sanity I couldn't afford to leave any stone unturned. Sadly, just as I thought the scan didn't harvest any of the answers I was looking for, the neurologist reported my scan to be 'normal with no irregularities'. On the plus side though

I was able to rule out brain tumours or anything particularly sinister.

After a whole two years had passed if anything my tinnitus had only grown worse, although it would be fair to say after sort of accepting it wasn't going away, I had learned a little better to live with tinnitus rather than to fight it. In stubborn defiance the buzzing had progressed to new extremes. It had evolved to impact on the basic day-to-day noises, conversations, traffic, music and general background noise. My Tinnitus was no longer a problem just in silence it was now a problem it almost every environment, noise or no noise. After a pretty bleak introduction to this book, it would be entirely understandable to feel a little deflated but please stick with me and the good news is this cloud does have a silver lining!

If you are reading this and suffer with tinnitus it is likely to be much easier for you to understand some the experiences I have described so far. However, for those of you who are fortunate enough to not suffer with tinnitus I hope this book helps you to appreciate the impact it can have on people's lives and those around them. Like a cancer the negative impact on my life continued to spread starting with my relationship, my marriage heavily deteriorated, the never-ending ringing would make me so anxious, agitated, impatient and tetchy, I have absolutely no doubt I had become a very difficult person to live with. The vicious circle of problems which included no sleep leading to over-tiredness, lack of concentration and general day-to-day brain fog. Inevitably this had worn me down and ultimately taken its toll and cost me my marriage. The words I write will never be enough to accurately describe how difficult tinnitus is to live with but regardless I will be doing my very best to help you both relate to me and understand what you are going through. It is often met with utter disbelief when I explain to people that the aggravating factor in my marriage failure was tinnitus, most people either roll their eyes or laugh, it those people who fail to understand the severity of this horrid condition. I do hope that some of those non-believers one day read this, maybe just maybe it will make a difference in their one-dimensional opinions, I won't hold my breath.

Throughout the last few years, I have experienced both high and low-pitched tinnitus, from reading countless articles on the subject I appear to have had the platinum package - the full range of tinnitus. Sadly, there were some knock-on diagnoses and conditions I experienced which I can directly link to having tinnitus. It wasn't long before I was clinically diagnosed with depression and extreme anxiety, this led to me becoming terribly reclusive I would hunch over at the thought of a social event and would voluntarily exclude myself from anything like this.

I associate a great deal of importance to telling you what I went through, by doing this hopefully you and me can build an understanding. I absolutely need you know I have the highest amount of sympathy for what you are currently going through as a sufferer or a family member of a sufferer. As part of my quest to cure my own condition I have researched the impact of tinnitus sufferers globally, I have studied the symptoms of hundreds of tinnitus patients and read and researched all known cures. I have weighed up the pros and cons of all and been a human Guinee-pig for almost everything available to tinnitus sufferers, ultimately out of pure desperation. You are reading this book from somebody who understands this subject inside out as a sufferer and a student of the condition, I really hope that helps you to be able to relate to me. However bad your tinnitus may-be I truly want you to know that despite all of this there is hope and I believe you can be cured or at the very least make big strides to help you manage your tinnitus and make significant improvements. The good news is you won't have to go to the other side of the world to get it, in fact you may not have to travel very far at all, hopefully all the answers and solutions will be right here before you in this book.

Do you remember what silence feels like? Or is it all just a distant memory. Until you suffer with tinnitus, I guess it's just another one of those things in life which we take for granted. Silence is a truly blissful treasure and one of life's gifts one that I never appreciated before but I definitely do now.   I can remember wondering if I would ever experience silence again, I thought my days of silence were truly long gone and would never live to experience another blissfully silent moment again. Perhaps you can take a little bit of hope from the fact that I was once again able to experience it and as a matter of fact I still do, hopefully, in time after benefiting from the instructions in this book you can once again experience that too.

Chapter 1

The School of Google

I am not a supernatural mind reader nor do I possess any remote kind of mystical powers but there is one thing I know about you. I can almost certainly guarantee that prior to reading this book you have become a devoted student of 'The School of Google'. Go on, tell me I am wrong I dare you! You have been found out, it's ok, your secret is safe with me. How could I or anyone else possibly criticise you for allowing yourself with a little google self-diagnostics, after all haven't, we all graduated from the university of Google? I am certainly guilty. Of-course as you have probably guessed I am not going to spend any time encouraging you to do this. The dangers of google diagnosis is that although many snippets of information may well be correct, many pieces of information will certainly be incorrect. It's 2023, and the default reaction to most problems are consult Dr

Google. Even though it is such a powerful search engine it will not discriminate between right and wrong, the paid adverts are almost always near the top, naturally the ads (some helpful) are money making schemes or huge corporate web-based giants. Googling becomes a filtration process, this subject in particular can lead you on many a wild goose chase, ultimately, I am not advising you to never do this, but for goodness's sake please be really careful.

When my ears began to ring consistently for more than 24 hours my first port of call was not the GP, not to consult books written on the subject or a tinnitus specialist, of course it was our trust friend again – Dr Google! Looking back, I now know this was counter-productive, after just few clicks of my mouse I was reading bespoke scaremongering literature such as 'tinnitus is for life', 'there is no cure for tinnitus', 'my tinnitus never went away' 'It's linked to tumours' 'Tinnitus is a sign of Cancer'. Given that over 60% of all tinnitus sufferers believe that the condition was triggered by stress, anxiety and depression. I cannot fathom why anyone serious about helping on the subject would publish such negative rubbish. So perhaps the first tip in this book is to guide you away from googling yourself into a tinnitus tis. Assuming you have already consulted google and you have lost all hope of a cure, you have come to the right place as there is hope and everything is possible. I want to show you some methods that will undoubtably help you and in some cases cure your tinnitus entirely.

During your own research you may have also read about the possibility of surgery to correct your tinnitus, my lengthy research suggests this is an increasingly popular option especially in the U.S.A, there are many arguments for and against. There has been much written on this and the evidence points towards surgery being a successful cure option, but like all surgery it comes with risk. We will cover this on more detail in the book and allow you to make your own mind up, with Tinnitus comes desperation and in turn I understand that all options remain in play for you. Personally, I believe in an alternative strategy in the form of 9 Key steps which I will educate you on shortly. It's easy for me to say do this or don't do that but in fairness I do consider myself to self-cured - without surgery. In the next chapter we I will go into some detail about what actually causes tinnitus, if we are to concur it, we must first understand it so your attention and patience is appreciated.

Chapter 2

What Causes Tinnitus?

Although I strongly believe all Tinnitus sufferers are very different my own research suggests that there are a number of common denominations when it comes to the causes. The more people I have spoken too, the more I have read have all led me to a list of aggravating causes which are as follows. As you read through the below list try and answer in your head if any of the below triggers apply to you (that you are aware of)

Key Tinnitus triggers

Stress - Are you stressed? Do you feel stressed? Allot going on in your life? This can be a huge contributing factor to tinnitus.

Caffeine – Do you drink to much Tea, Coffee or energy drinks? If you do notice how this effects your tinnitus symptoms.

Clogged arteries around the middle ear or inner ear – A doctor or the ENT department should quickly be able to establish if this is the cause.

Anaemia - Very common cause. Basically, Anaemia is your body not having enough healthy red blood cells.

Prolonged exposure to loud sounds – Do you currently or have you worked in an aloud industrial environment, pubs, nightclubs? Exposure to excessive noise is proven to cause long term damage to hearing and resulting in Tinnitus.

Age - common after 55 years of age are you older or younger than 55?

Gender - Men are 35% more likely prone to suffer from tinnitus.

Smoking – Another thing to add to the never-ending list of reasons not to smoke.

Cardiovascular disease – Get your cholesterol, blood pressure checked, find out if cardiovascular disease runs in the family. If you are worried it could be this then its wise to seek professional medical advice

High blood pressure – Definitely check if your BP is operating at normal healthy levels by visiting your GP.

Overactive thyroid – Establish this again via GP, a simple blood test referral will establish this.

Underactive thyroid – Again blood test will tell all.

Tumours in head and neck – Doctors should quickly be able to eliminate or diagnose this as the cause and establish if there are any more severe related health concerns.

Coronavirus - The newest addition to the symptom list. Covid-19 has meant more tinnitus sufferers have been diagnosed than ever before, Covid-19 has now been formally recognised by the BTA (British Tinnitus Association) as a recognised cause of the illness.

How do you know you have Tinnitus?

Tinnitus symptoms can vary significantly from person to person. You may hear phantom sounds in one ear, in both ears and in your head. The phantom sound may ring, buzz, roar, whistle, hum, click, hiss, or squeak. The sounds may be softish or loud and may vary from high pitched and low pitched. It may come and go or in some cases be present all the time. Sometimes by moving your head, neck, or eyes, or touching certain parts of your body may produce tinnitus symptoms or temporarily change the quality of the perceived sound. This is called somatosensory (pronounced so-ma-toe-SENSE-uh-ree) tinnitus.

The majority of tinnitus are entirely *subjective*, meaning that only you can hear the sounds. In more unusual cases, the sound seemingly creates a pulsating rhythmical sensation, often in time to your heartbeat. In these particular cases, a doctor may be able to hear the sounds with a stethoscope and, if so, it is considered to be *objective* tinnitus. I experienced this when my tinnitus was at its most extreme. Often, objective tinnitus has an identifiable cause and is treatable. In many cases this is not detectable by a stethoscope which can be frustrating because nobody can actually hear what you are experiencing.

As a tinnitus sufferer it may well be that you suffer with one or more of the above listed symptoms, it may be that yours is caused by something entirely different. In this very early stage of the book, I have purposefully left the next couple of pages blank for your participation and self-reflection. Have you ever really sat and seriously pondered the possible causes of your tinnitus. Thinking about the common factors listed above please write down which ones you think apply to you and why. For example, prolonged exposure to loud sounds – Ask yourself did you spend all of your late teens and early twenties in extremely loud nightclubs? If so, how often and when? Try to put a date or a year on it, this will ultimately help when diagnoses and cures are on the agenda. Did you work on a building site with super noisy machinery? Do you still work on a building site with extremely loud machinery and go nightclubbing? It is really important to just take a moment to self-reflect at this stage of book as some people just don't realise the cause could have been quite obvious or consider the fact that they could even still be exposing themselves to an environment that is the cause or aggravating the symptoms. It's really key you get pen to paper at this juncture, I am certain this will be of help at a later stage. You should also consider the possibility of compensation, if you think your tinnitus was caused by a work place or a form of negligence then your accuracy in reflection will definitely help. When you do begin to write, please be as honest as you can with yourself, these are your notes, supporting your recovery and document your journey.

MY TINNITUS JOURNEY NOTES

Began End of may 2023
Head phones started wearing around 12th
Wore several hours at a time listening to Audible
Noticed ringing in my Ears around 20th-25th

Ringing has increased in Volume.
Its now been 8 weeks

Had Ear Test 12th July only loss is top end.

Cant sleep!
prescribed sleeping tablet 7th July.
Relaxation yoga Deep Breathing & Exercise.

Feeling Broken! Brain Fog
Focus gone misery.
General feeling unwell + Tired

Saw GP. Prescribed Antidepsants
and said it was Stress.

There is a lot going on in my life!

Hearing Test Proved that my
Hearing is ok just top Notes.
Sound like a Million Crickets
all at once

Sleeping Tablet have run out
using Alternative

Took only half of. Zoperclone

Diazapam Seems to Quiet it a bit
but Dont want to take offten.

Started to use my sleep Machine
again seem to help a bit.

Listen to Sounds of Rain and
Rolling thunder. Luna App

Cochlear
implants

Webinar.

Now about 11 - 12 weeks

Had Neck maniputation which
seemed to help a bit.
Suggested chewing menthol gum
magnesium an zinc added to Diet
Stopped Drinking coffee
doing breathing exercises
Put)menthol Under my Nose at night.

Noise Levels Vary.

Monitor Taking Valium or Diazpam
reduces the Volume But not Advisable

only take when really Tired.

I Dont Notice the Noise when Concentration
is involved
Didnt hear it when I took Pixie
to the vet.
Quite Places I stant to Listen again.
Thursday hardly Listen to it
During the Day
London good Day Didnt Notice too
Dont Hear when engaged   much
when on own in silence Loud

Nights still not good

Loud when [19] tired

CBT   EMDR
Consider?   Speak to GP

Chapter 3

What exactly is Tinnitus?

By its very definition tinnitus is described by the national institute of deafness and other communication issues (NIH) as the following;

Tinnitus (pronounced tih-NITE-us or TIN-uh-tus) is the perception of sound that does not have an external source, so other people cannot hear it. Tinnitus is commonly described as a ringing sound, but some people hear other types of sounds, such as roaring or buzzing. Tinnitus is common, with surveys estimating that 10 to 25% of adults have it. Children can also suffer with tinnitus. Children and adults' tinnitus may improve or even disappear over time, but in some cases, it worsens with time. When tinnitus lasts for three months or longer, it is considered chronic.

According the BTA, of the people who last saw their GP more than a year ago for tinnitus, incredibly only 2.4% say their treatment worked, while 46% believe 'there doesn't seem to be any point'. While the National Institute for Health and Care Excellence (NICE) introduced new guidance in 2021 to improve the care given for tinnitus, only 1.82% of respondents say this had a positive impact on their condition. How can the success rates be so low? It's now believed an effort by the NHS and other health bodies throughout the world are joining forced for a more collaborative effort to make improvements and ore funding is allegedly being allocated to deliver more research to 'collate medical, audiological and condition-specific information as well as biological samples, from people with tinnitus'. Either way the current results from medical intervention are just not good enough for 2023. Part of the reason for me writing this book was for exactly this reason, there appears to be very little help available from those who call themselves audiology professionals.

What actually creates the perception of noise inside the ears?

A commonly believed theory is that tinnitus can occur when damage to the inner ear modified the signals carried via the nerves to different parts to varying parts of the brain, usually toward areas in the brain which are designed to process sound. Potentially a good way to understand what is happening is to consider that while tinnitus may seem to occur in your ear, the phantom type sounds are in reality generated by your brain, in an area known as the auditory cortex, this is located on the temporal lobe situated on both sides of the brain.

Further evidence exists to suggest that unusual interactions between the auditory cortex and other neural circuitry plays a definitive role in causing tinnitus to begin. To explain the mechanics of this you need to understand the auditory cortex communicates with other parts of the brain, for example the area of your brain that control your attention and emotions. Some detailed research has indicated that some people with tinnitus have changes in these non-audible areas of the brain.

Auditory pathways of Tinnitus

Sound waves travel through the ear canal to the middle and inner ear, where hair cells in part of the cochlea help transform sound waves into electrical signals that then travel to the brain's auditory cortex via the auditory nerve. When hair cells are damaged —usually by loud noise or ingestion of ototoxic drugs, for example, the circuits in the brain then stop receive the signals they're expecting. This stimulates abnormal activity in the neurons, which results in the illusion of sound, or tinnitus being created. Trying to get your head around the science of it is enough to trigger tinnitus alone, I hope by explaining the mechanics I haven't stressed you out too much. I think key to understand what is happening, without doubt expanding my understanding at the beginning was integral to beginning a journey of self-improvement

What is actually going on inside?

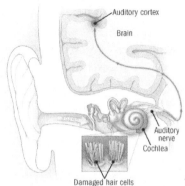

This illustration perfectly captures the mechanics of the link between the inner ear and auditory cortex

How is tinnitus best diagnosed?

As I have already explained I have followed a common journey in my own diagnoses. In the interests of your own generic health and to eliminate any further sinister issues I would highly recommend you first see your GP, who will usually check for a build-up of earwax or fluid from any recent ear infections that could be blocking your ear canal. It is likely your doctor will also discuss with you your medical history to find out if an underlying condition or a medication may be causing your tinnitus.

Next, you may be likely be referred to an otolaryngologist (commonly called an ear, nose, and throat doctor, or an ENT). If your doctor is reluctant to refer you it is important you are insistent upon this. ENTs are generally a very busy part of the hospital and frequently oversubscribed. I am not suggesting this will be the reason behind the reluctance to refer but do not let this put you off. Again, due to ENT's being over-subscribed it can sometimes take many months to even get an initial appointment, if this is the case and financially viable for you, please consider the option of a private ENT consultation, by doing this you will skip the waiting times and quite possibly get better service in general. The ENT will inevitably ask you to describe the tinnitus symptoms you are experiencing in detail and will also want to know when they first started, remember this is where the notes section may come in handy. ENT will examine your head, neck, and ears in great detail. You might also be further referred to an audiologist, who can measure your hearing and evaluate your tinnitus. Audiology testing is an extremely thorough examination that can last up to two hours and during this appointment you will undergo a series of detailed inner ear function tests. During my own experience I have used national heath service ENT's & Audiologists and indeed both specialists in the private sector. A word of warning if you do intend to do this privately then these appointments can be incredibly costly, luckily for me I had private health care before my official diagnoses which covered this for me but to give you an idea of cost; Private health audiologist appointments can be £1000+ ($1300).

The ENT and audiology department may consider ordering imaging tests, especially if your tinnitus gives you a pulsating sensation. Imaging tests such as magnetic resonance imaging (MRI), computed tomography (CT), or ultrasound can help reveal whether a structural problem or underlying medical condition is causing your tinnitus.

CHAPTER 4

Experiences shared

By now you should have a deeper understanding of how tinnitus works, you will hopefully have related to my self-declared credentials of being a genuine sufferer. In my experience I have always found it more suitable to learn from those who have genuinely experienced a problem rather than somebody who has just studied the subject. I felt it important to spend a significant portion of this book building that rapport with you before we begin to take some significantly effective steps to help you.

There are over a 300 million world-wide diagnosed sufferers of this illness all with variant levels of severity and my goal is to reach out to of many of you as possible. It is possible that along your tinnitus journey you may have felt such extreme levels of frustration that you felt beyond all help and as a result been in complete despair. It wouldn't be unusual for tinnitus to have triggered depression and in extreme cases and God forbid – suicidal thoughts. If you have felt any of the above you certainly would not be alone in feeling like this. I for one have had these feelings before things got better for me. You need to be aware that no matter how bad things are for you, things can and will get better, the situation will improve even if it is just choosing to accept it. I fully expect only tinnitus sufferers or former tinnitus sufferers like me will really feel understand your sufferance, might find sharing this kind of problem a little more niche that most other things but trust me there is a whole lot of support available starting with right here. There are 100's of online forums out there, a simple online search won't require you to look very far at all to find them, forums are a good place to share your experience and talk through the problems with others that understand it. I have to say this but if you really are at the end of your own personal coping limit and are feeling anything like suicidal then this is something you should definitely share with friends, family and more urgently a GP, those thoughts and feelings should never be harboured alone.

You absolutely need to know that you are not alone and there is certain hope for you, whatever you do please don't feel isolated. Just to hammer home the point let's take a look at two other people just like you and me in two real life and very typical tinnitus suffering examples.

Case Study One

For tinnitus sufferer Peter from, a 48-year-old from Bolton, Lancashire, he highlights just one of the reasons why tinnitus frequently affects his mental health and wellbeing, he explains 'I was unable to function in normal daily activities, could not socialise and couldn't be around my family due to noise sensitivity. 'I felt very shut off from the world with no one to help and know cure known. 'You can't shut the sound of tinnitus off, it's there 24/7. Feelings of anger, loneliness, helplessness and fear were very real. 'Peter was officially diagnosed in November 2019 after working it out for himself a few months earlier. He explained: 'I pretty much had to self-diagnose. 'I was waiting for such a long time for the NHS due to waiting lists and lack, there appeared to be a real lack of knowledge that I researched as much as I could which led me to the BTA. 'It was only when I went to a private doctor, around three months after the onset, that he told me I had most likely hyperacusis alongside tinnitus.' Since then, he has tried therapy and a hearing aid that was designed to reduce noise levels. Peter says the early stages of having tinnitus are especially difficult to manage, as you're hyperaware of the condition. 'For the first few months, it's no lie, it impacts on 100% of the day's focus,' he says. 'You listen to see if it is louder, quieter, or if it has changed in pitch or tone. 'Over a year later, with the management techniques I have learned from my own research and understanding, I would say it is noticeable around 20% of my day – mainly due to work stress or my kids when they are being noisy.'

According to the British Tinnitus Association (BTA), the number of tinnitus cases in the UK alone could exceed half a million over the next 5-10 years – especially that now it's a recognised symptom of Long Covid. In many cases, people have likened the sound they hear to 'a high-pitched hiss', 'screaming' or 'like a pressure cooker going off'.

Case Study Two

Dannielle Taylor-Robertson from Bethnal Green, London has suffered with tinnitus for three years. She's just 28, which proves it can come into a person's life at any time. After being formally diagnosed, she explains she was told: 'The best thing to do was to just live with it. 'She says: 'I really felt disheartened and thought "How can I live with this condition? It is absolutely destroying my life". I felt really let down and started to become depressed. 'When I got the diagnosis, I was scared and started to research it, this was a dangerous game as there are many rabbit holes in using internet search engines to try and find solutions to problems. This really stressed me out. 'Tinnitus felt like torture and my mental health was destroyed' 'My stress and tinnitus became a toxic vicious cycle where my tinnitus made me feel stressed and my stress exacerbated the tinnitus worse. 'In the first three months it affected my mental health drastically. 'Tinnitus felt like torture and my mental health was destroyed. 'One day I was walking with my mum and told her that did want to live anymore. It must be every parent's worst nightmare to hear, but I really felt that bad.' At her worst, tinnitus is on her mind constantly. At her best, it's something she only consciously thinks about when hearing a high-pitched noise. No treatment that's currently available has worked for Danielle, so she's gone down the holistic healing route to relieve her symptoms. 'I have had physiotherapy and reflexology and I feel so much better now than I did. 'I have been able to reframe tinnitus in my mind and I feel much more in control,' she added.

CHAPTER 5

Tinnitus Cures & Making life easier

Congratulations, you have reached the part of the book you have been waiting for, the part where we get to the nitty gritty and seriously talk about solutions to this horrendous condition, at the very least if we can't ultimately formulate a permanent cure for you then I certainly remain confident that you will be making some comfortable improvements to how you cope day-to-day with tinnitus. I do completely admire those of you who had the foresight and wisdom to bypass the introductory stages of this book. If you are one of the page skipping individuals then of-course your time saving is completely fine by me, however I must recommend (if time will allow) you do go back and read the chapters leading up to this part of the book. I truly believe this will maximise your chances of sticking with the forthcoming solutions for a sustainable period of time.

Within this chapter I will be sharing with you my collective secrets of how I healed myself. I don't think I have mentioned up until now but it might be encouraging for you to know that I am no longer a tinnitus sufferer, that's right, against all the odds I have made the transition back into what I previously understood to be 'normality', subsequently I am now fully able to embrace the sheer luxury of silence like never before. My methods have worked wonders for me and many others but be aware that an accumulative invested approach is required for you to gain the full benefits of my recommended steps, as my late father used to say 'Nothing changes unless something changes'. I have coined that phrase many times since and the more I have used it and thought about it over the years the more I have come to know just how that that is. In other words, in order to harvest massive results - you have to put in massive action. Over the last couple of decades, I have read and digested practically all of the self-help books the the library has to offer, within the hundreds of books, papers and articles digested I have learned one underlining theme that reoccurs in so many books -**Timing is everything!** Allow me to explain, you need to be **ready** to commit to a change. You have invested your money and your time in this book, therefore it's my duty to be honest with you. Picking up a book, reading or watching a video on YouTube is one thing, action and reaction to a problem or making a change is another. One thing is certain you are not going to cure your tinnitus by doing nothing, so you need to act and in order to act you need to be ready to aggressively act. It is scientifically recognised that it takes 21 days to form a habit, I personally believe it is longer than that so be prepared for a slightly longer haul. The time in your life to make lasting changes are best achieved when you have minimal distraction, taking on too much will most likely hinder rather than help. So, what I am trying to say is; if you are the middle of buying a new house, having a baby, trying to recover from a nervous breakdown, gunning for a big promotion at work or anything that is going to consume the best of your energy then I would urge you to come back to the action steps of this book at a later date when you are ready to fully commit. This ethos is especially poignant to this particular condition as we both know tinnitus is typically aggravated by stress and having too much on your plate at one time. My absolute goal is to help you achieve the very best results and to do that you need to be ready and in the right frame of mind.

Just before we begin, I am going to anticipate a few burning questions you may have regarding the cure process. How long is this going to take? The answer to this varies from person to person and the level of commitment you are able to apply. Typically, within 40 days you should be feeling remarkably better and notice a significant improvement. Between 40 days and 60 days you could potentially be cured indefinitely. Of course, I am not in a position to offer any god like guarantees on your health, every single one of us are different, none the less I am very confident you have every chance of complete success. You have already taken a massive step, you found this book, you are taking the time to read this book, this truly means that if nothing else you want to help yourself and above all things you have yet to give up hope. Give yourself a massive pat on the back and congratulate yourself as you are now truly on the correct path.

The guidance steps listed below are carefully written in the order I have found to be most productive and effective, however it would be unproductive of me to set in stone any hard and fast rules as to in which order you should apply them to yourself as each case of tinnitus is different, we all have different lifestyles and commitments and for the reason I would advise you to apply them in the order that seems to be more accommodating to your lifestyle. At the end of the book, I will add a quick reference list for you to follow, which may save you from having to come back and read chapter after chapter.

Without any further ado, let us begin.

Step 1 Introducing Breathing, Relaxation & Calmness

Breathing is the first crucial step in your pathway to recovery. How often do you think about your breathing? Does your breathing require any thinking or does it just happen? The answer is of course it just happens, generally speaking we just breath without applying any conscious thoughts at all. Breathing is governed by our autonomic nervous system better understood as our bodily auto-pilot which operates the basic survival functions without the requirement to think or process information. The autonomic nervous system also manages our digestive system, circulation, fights infection, filters blood and hundreds of other amazing functions which when you begin to look closely will blow your mind. The human body is an amazingly resilient well-designed piece of kit, surprisingly robust and completely regenerative. In-fact did you know your cells completely regenerate over a 10-year period meaning essentially that in 10 years you are quite literally an entirely different person. You should be encouraged by the frequency of cell regeneration, since cells are regenerated so frequently this also means nerves which make up the audible cortex in the brain are also regenerated, what if that particular set of cells regenerated in perfect working order and functionality? Is that possible? I certainly believe so. The key core function of our body is primarily regulated by our breathing and if we learn to breath in the right way we can begin to achieve so much more and importantly feel so much better. Regulated, focussed and concentrated breathing can initiate a whole host of positive tigger health benefits for our bodies, not least the stimulation of healing processes. By collaborating focussed breathing activities with a positive dedicated mind-set, you will highly likely experience quite tangible bodily functional improvement.

The mind body and soul can be fully revitalised by regular intervals of focussed, timely breathing leading to a positive shift in your neuro-transmitional profile which is conveniently and directly linked to the functionality of the audible cortex, this is the area which we now know your tinnitus originates. This isn't a book about spiritual healing but there is some very strong evidence that focussed breathing and putting yourself into semi mediative states can be incredibly powerful and there is hard evidence to suggest significant health improvements a result. As I have begun to explore further and further down the rabbit whole of spiritual and holistic healing, I have procured one certain fact which I truly believe helps the in the fight against tinnitus - Focussed breathing.

From day to day how much do you truly think about your breathing? Be honest, do you ever consider your breathing and practice any form of relaxation exercise? The answer is probably no, the 21st century high paced lifestyle doesn't allow for it. The moments where we historically spent in wind down mode have now been replaced by smart phones and other mentally stimulating interactive devices which constantly activate our brains far more than they are designed to accommodate. Sleep, relaxation and rejuvenation are fundamental to our genetic make-up and are key players in supporting optimum day to day functionality in the mind, body and soul. Too many of us are rejecting the opportunity to allow our bodies to do this and subsequently illnesses like tinnitus are rapidly increasing.

So, your first step on the road to cured tinnitus starts here which means you need to make a small self-investment at this stage and it starts by allowing for 3 ten-minute intervals per day (completely away from whatever you are doing). By planning intervals and re-programming your mind to adhere to it you will be manifesting some unbelievable progress. I found this hard at first with such a busy lifestyle but I learned to use a technique called habit stacking.

Go somewhere quiet, preferably where there are no other people, this could be your car, another room, somewhere where you can sit comfortably with your head back and relax your head and shoulders.

1) As we know silence can be the enemy so if you wish and it helps put on some headphones and play some gentle music, sounds of nature waves crashing etc.

2) When you are completely comfortable close your eyes gently and begin to take deep breaths in through the nose, let the air filter way down in the bottom of your core and if you are able hold for a couple of seconds before breathing slowly out through your mouth, all the way out until the tummy has flattened and the air has vacated your diaphragm. Repeat this process, be sure to breath all the way in, all the way out slowly. As you do

this, I want you to think about your breathing and breathing only, think about the oxygen filling your blood, think about it circulating around your veins, into your arms legs, and organs. Imagine the oxygen replenishing the cells in your brain and revitalising your thoughts. Just focus on the breathing and think only of the breathing. If another thought does enter your mind, this is normal, allow if but let it slowly drift away before gently refocussing on the breathing. Continue to repeat this process for around 20-30 times until you begin to feel completely relaxed.

3) As you enter the feeling of deeper relaxation and remove yourself from the stresses of your day-to-day activities, I now want you to think about you eye lids and only your eyelids. Imagine them being the heaviest part of your body, so heavy that no matter how hard you try you cannot open them. Begin to count from one to ten, still breathing gently and on each number your eye lids are feeling heavier, no matter how hard you try your eyes are closed and can't be opened until you have decided that your body has entered a feeling of complete and total relaxation. Just for a short while now hold this feeling while maintaining steady, concentrated breathing before gently counting down from ten to one, this time with each count and each breath you are now steadily becoming more and more awake.

Your arms, legs, body and mind are gently coming back to life.

4) When you have finished the count slowly open your eyes and just take a moment to acknowledge you, your body, your soul, how lucky you are, the good things you have in life and how good you feel in the moment!

5) Slowly sit yourself up and continue you with your day.

6) Don't forget you now need to come back and repeat this process on two more occasions in the same day. As the days go on and you must do this like a religion, just like the habitual day-to-day tasks such as showering, getting dressed & drinking a cup of coffee. Within just a couple of weeks this will then become a habit. When you begin to realise how much better you are feeling from doing this simple step at the cost of less than 1% of your day this will also then become an essential process and in time you may even be doing this without thinking about it. This wont just help you with curing tinnitus it will help improve breathing, self-relaxation and bring an abundance of other health benefits.

The above six steps are my own bespoke breathing plan which worked for me. As I have illuded too many times in this book - we are all different, you have to do what works for you. For that reason, I have detailed a list of well-known successful breathing techniques, all or any

38

of the techniques I have shown should all have the same desired effect so please feel free to use any of the patterns described in any combination. All I ask and hope is that you commit to finding the time and space to doing this 3 times a daily, especially at the start of your journey.

Alternate-Nostril Breathing

Alternate-nostril breathing (*nadi shodhana*) involves blocking off one nostril at a time as you breathe through the other, alternating between nostrils in a regular pattern. It's best to practice this type of anxiety-relieving breathing in a seated position in order to maintain your posture.

- Position your right hand by bending your pointer and middle fingers into your palm, leaving your thumb, ring finger, and pinky extended. This is known as *Vishnu mudra* in yoga.
- Close your eyes or softly gaze downward.
- Inhale and exhale to begin.
- Close off your right nostril with your thumb.
- Inhale through your left nostril.
- Close off your left nostril with your ring finger.
- Open and exhale through your right nostril.
- Inhale through your right nostril.

- Close off your right nostril with your thumb.
- Open and exhale through your left nostril.
- Inhale through your left nostril.

Work up to 10 rounds of this breathing pattern. If you begin to feel lightheaded, take a break by releasing both nostrils and breathing normally.

Belly Breathing

According to The American Institute of Stress, 20 to 30 minutes of "belly breathing," also known as abdominal breathing or diaphragmatic breathing, each day can reduce stress and anxiety

Find a comfortable, quiet place to sit or lie down. For example, try sitting in a chair, sitting cross-legged, or lying on your back with a small pillow under your head and another under your knees.

- Place one hand on your upper chest and the other hand on your belly, below the ribcage.
- Allow your belly to relax, without forcing it inward by squeezing or clenching your muscles.
- Breathe in slowly through your nose. The air should move into your nose and downward so that you feel your stomach rise with your other hand and fall inward (toward your spine).

40

- Exhale slowly through slightly pursed lips. Take note of the hand on your chest, which should remain relatively still.

Box Breathing

Also known as four-square breathing, **box breathing** is very simple to learn and practice. In fact, if you've ever noticed yourself inhaling and exhaling to the rhythm of a song, you're already familiar with this type of paced breathing. It goes like this:

- Exhale to a count of four.
- Hold your lungs empty for a four-count.
- Inhale to a count of four.
- Hold the air in your lungs for a count of four.
- Exhale and begin the pattern anew.

4-7-8 Breathing

The 4-7-8 breathing exercise, also called the relaxing breath, acts as a natural tranquilizer for the nervous system. At first, it's best to perform the exercise seated with your back straight. Once you become more familiar with this breathing exercise, however, you can perform it while lying in bed.

- Place and keep the tip of your tongue against the ridge of tissue behind your upper front teeth for the duration of the exercise.
- Completely exhale through your mouth, making a "whoosh" sound.
- Close your mouth and inhale quietly through your nose to a mental count of four.
- Hold your breath for a count of seven.
- Exhale completely through your mouth, making a whoosh sound to a count of eight.

Lion's Breath

Lion's breath, or *simhasana* in Sanskrit, during which you stick out your tongue and roar like a lion, is another helpful deep breathing practice. It can help relax the muscles in your face and jaw, alleviate stress, and improve cardiovascular function.

The exercise is best performed in a comfortable, seated position, leaning forward slightly with your hands on your knees or the floor.

- Spread your fingers as wide as possible.
- Inhale through your nose.
- Open your mouth wide, stick out your tongue, and stretch it down toward your chin.

- Exhale forcefully, carrying the breath across the root of your tongue.
- While exhaling, make a "ha" sound that comes from deep within your abdomen.
- Breathe normally for a few moments.
- Repeat lion's breath up to seven times.

Mindfulness Breathing

Mindfulness meditation involves focusing on your breathing and bringing your attention to the present without allowing your mind to drift to the past or future. Engaging in mindfulness breathing exercises serves the same purpose, which can help ease your anxiety.

One mindfulness breathing exercise to try involves choosing a calming focus, including a sound ("om"), positive word ("peace"), or phrase ("breathe in calm, breathe out tension") to repeat silently as you inhale or exhale. Let go and relax. If you notice that your mind has drifted, take a deep breath and gently return your attention to the present.

Pursed-Lip Breathing

Pursed-lip breathing is a simple breathing technique that will help make deep breaths slower and more intentional. This technique has been found to benefit people who have anxiety associated with lung conditions like emphysema and chronic obstructive pulmonary disease (COPD).

- Sit in a comfortable position with your neck and shoulders relaxed.
- Keeping your mouth closed, inhale slowly through your nostrils for two seconds.
- Exhale through your mouth for four seconds, puckering your lips as if giving a kiss.
- Keep your breath slow and steady while breathing out.

To get the correct breathing pattern, experts recommend practicing pursed-lip breathing four to five times a day.

Resonance Breathing

Resonance breathing, or coherent breathing, can help you get into a relaxed state and reduce anxiety.

1. Lie down and close your eyes.
2. Gently breathe in through your nose, mouth closed, for a count of six seconds. Don't fill your lungs too full of air.
3. Exhale for six seconds, allowing your breath to leave your body slowly and gently without forcing it.
4. Continue for up to 10 minutes.
5. Take a few additional minutes to be still and focus on how your body feels.

Simple Breathing Exercises

You can perform this simple breathing exercise as often as needed. It can be done standing up, sitting, or lying down. If you find this exercise difficult or believe it's making you anxious or panicky, stop for now. Try it again in a day or so and build up the time gradually.

1. Inhale slowly and deeply through your nose. Keep your shoulders relaxed. Your abdomen should expand, and your chest should rise very little.
2. Exhale slowly through your mouth. As you blow air out, purse your lips slightly but keep your jaw relaxed. You may hear a soft "whooshing" sound as you exhale.
3. Repeat this breathing exercise. Do it for several minutes until you start to feel better.

When you chose this book, you may have not expected to stumble across a few pages of guidance around breathing, I guess you are going to have to trust me on this. Hopefully the comprehensive choice of breathing exercises listed will provide you at least one pattern that works for you. I fully expect the hardest part to be finding the time, motivation to actually do it and most importantly stick to it. I urge you to give it a try at the very least though, it is by no coincidence that I have listed this right at the top of my cure guidance.

STEP 2 – Electromagnetic devices & Bluescreen exposure

I guess time is yet to tell if mobile phones and other portable electronic devices are detrimental to our long-term health. I have developed my own theory on this subject as I believe mobile phones can be our best friend and also our worst enemy, I personally believe (although please note not scientifically proven) that excessive phone exposure directly effects tinnitus. Way back in the 1920's,30s & 40's almost 85% of all adults were smokers, why is this? Mainly because people simply weren't aware of the dangers that existed caused by inhaling tar, nicotine and many other toxins directly into our lungs. Around this difficult period in history, it's easy to understand how adults turned to smoking as one of the very few enjoyments in life to distract them from the troubles and trauma of World Wars 1 &2. Would 85% of adults have smoked if they knew then what we know now? Over a number of decades, we have suffered monumental increases of cancer diagnoses, many of those have been directly linked to smoking. As medical science has enhanced, we have become much more aware of the dangers that exist and therefore the adult population smoking statistics have subsequently fallen dramatically. That figure is now more like 15% in the western cultures like US & UK.

I first started using a mobile phone way back in 1997, my first contract was with a UK service network provider. Upon signing up for my first contract I got my hands on a shiny new Nokia 5210. It was life changing in so many ways. As part of the many benefits gifted to me from this fantastic new device, I was gifted 50 minutes of talk time per day to any other orange user or UK landline, boy did I take advantage of that. I remember calling people just for the sake of it. At the time I wasn't aware of any dangers linked to the use of putting a mobile device directly to my ear, fast forward to 2023 and the general population are still not wholly aware on how this could impact us long term. However, within the last few years we have just begun to see the repercussions of long-term mobile phone use and direct links to hearing problems as a result. UAMS audiologist Dr. Allison Catlett Woodall says '" cell phone use exceeding 60 minutes per day could result in lasting damage such as high frequency hearing loss". If you suffer with high frequency hearing loss, this means generally speaking you are unable to hear sounds ranging from 2,000 to 8,000 Hertz, basically this means that there is a likelihood it may affect your ability to understand speech and discern consonants.

A separate study was also conducted by the American Academy of Otolaryngology which went some way to prove that the electromagnetic waves emitted by the phone caused lasting damage and that this hearing loss is not necessarily caused by the high volume. We are also now seeing out first law suits against mobile phone companies for failing to advice and protect its customers, as time goes on, we can only guess how serious this could become.

In the mean-time I don't want this part of the book to become about mobile phone scaremongering. There are many separate books and studies that could bore you for hours which highlight all of the possibilities. However, what I do what to do is get you thinking about this as a possibility. Based on my own experiences with mobile phones I have to confess that I have felt my ears heat up and literally heard and felt the buzzing, vibration and the electromagnetic waves zapping around inside my head (maybe I was being paranoid). Let me be very clear – I believe my own conscious effort to reduce mobile usage has positively impacted on my Tinnitus cure journey. I would like to point out I still use my smart phone every day, oh my god how could I be without it? but there are some significant adjustments which I made as to how I use it. If you want to follow my advice, I fully recommend you follow these mobile phone using steps.

1) Never take your phone to bed with you. If you do insist on doing so, make sure you switch it off and leave it on charge. By leaving your phone elsewhere in the house you will be reducing your direct electromagnetic transition exposure by around 8 hours. While we sleep our mind, body and soul repairs and moving the phone away is a wonderful opportunity of giving your head a

good rest, although this is just one benefit. Having the phone in the bedroom is a bad idea for so many reasons and another of those reasons is blue light exposure on the eyes before sleep, this is proven to negatively impact on falling asleep. Another major factor you need to be aware of is 'over stimulation of the mind'. By having the phone next to you it is likely that before sleep you will want to use it last thing before sleep and also presents the temptation to be the first thing you do when your eyes open. As hard as this might seem this is a hugely positive step. By making mobile phone use in the bedroom a non-event you will undoubtably reap the benefits and bring yourself another step closer to curing your tinnitus.

2) When you make or receive a call on your mobile phone try using a Bluetooth headset. By doing this you are once again you are reducing your electromagnetic exposure dramatically.

3) If you don't have a Bluetooth headset and prefer not to use them, try using the speakerphone option where ever possible.

4) Try making more use of the many other communication techniques, text, email, or even video conferencing which are now so readily accessible instead of talking on the phone or even more outrageously, here's an idea - how about a face-to-face conversation!

BLUE-SCREEN Awareness

I touched on this above but I would like to go into a little more detail on this subject. I am hoping you may have some baseline knowledge on the impact of blue-light exposure has on sleep ultimately leading to insomnia. There a many-studies linked to blue-screens negatively impacting on human sleep cycles. My personal opinion, once again based on my own experience is that a lack of sleep had a definite aggravating effect on my tinnitus, therefore I think its important we at least afford this subject the credence it deserves, so let us dig into the blue screen conundrum in a little more detail. Below I want to help you to understand how blue screens can become problematic and provide some step-by-step guidance on how to implement those changes on your tech.

The screen on your mobile device or computer normally emits a blue light that's fine for daytime use but can disrupt your sleep at night. That's because blue light stimulates your brain and fools it into thinking it's daytime, potentially keeping you awake if you use your device before bedtime.

While several studies have found that blue light can hinder your sleep, other studies have found the impact to be minimal, at least in small doses. With the data still inconclusive, limiting your exposure before bedtime is still worth trying, especially if you have difficulty falling asleep.

Your iPhone, iPad, and Windows PC have a feature called Night Shift for changing the colour temperature of the screen. Many Android devices also offer a built-in blue light filter, while a variety of third-party utility apps get the job done, too. Here's how to control the blue light on your device.

On your iPhone or iPad, go to **Settings > Display & Brightness**. Tap the **Night Shift** setting, which alters your screen to display colours of a warmer colour temperature, filtering out blue light.

You can set Night Shift to go on and off at predetermined times by turning on the **Scheduled** switch and setting a start time and end time for when the colour change should take effect. For example, you can set it to turn on an hour or so before you typically go to sleep and turn it off when you usually wake up.

Turn on **Manually Enable Until Tomorrow** to temporarily activate the blue light filter now until the start of the next day.

Night Shift can also be set specifically for Sunset to Sunrise, but if you don't see that option, go to **Settings > Privacy > Location Services > System Services** and turn on the Setting Time Zone option. Return to the Night Shift settings screen and tap the scheduled times. You'll now see the option for Sunset to Sunrise.

Use the slider to make the screen's colouring warmer or cooler. Warmer settings are best if you want to get a good night's sleep, but you'll want to find a balance so the screen is pleasing to view. Play around with this setting until you find the right temperature for you.

You can also turn on Night Shift mode from the Control Centre on your iPhone or iPad. Depending on the device you own, open Control Centre by swiping your finger up from the bottom of the screen or down from the top-right corner. Press down on the **Brightness** control, then tap the **Night Shift** button to turn it on.

Night Light / Blue Light Filter on Android Device

Most Android devices should have built-in blue light filters that can be enabled or disabled from the Settings screen. However, the feature's availability and options depend on your specific device and version of Android. You should be able to find the filter under **Settings > Display**. Look for an option for Night Light or Blue Light filter and turn it on.

In most cases there should be a way to schedule the feature and adjust the colour temperature to your liking. Scheduling it to turn on and off will be under the Schedule option, while an Intensity or Opacity option will let you change the colour temperature.

Blue-Light Filter Android Apps

If your Android device doesn't have a built-in Blue Light feature or doesn't have all the features you'd like, try one of several third-party apps that filter out blue light.

Blue Light Filter: The app allows you to easily adjust the colour temperature by choosing from among several pre-set options. The app even provides tips on the best temperature to make sure you fall asleep as you would normally. You can also tweak the intensity and the brightness of the filter.

sFilter: This app allows you to manually turn on a blue light filter or schedule it to turn on and off at specific times of the day or night. You can change the colour, opacity, and brightness of the filter. You can even create a shortcut icon or widget, so you don't have to open the app to enable the filter.

Twilight: The app advises you on the right colour temperature as you move a slider. Set the filter to always be enabled, run from sunrise to sunset, or turn on and off at specific times.

Night Light on Windows 10 or 11 Devices

If you use a Windows 10 or Windows 11 device before bedtime, you can bump into the same trouble trying to catch a good night's sleep. But Microsoft's Night Light feature can paint the screen with a warmer colour. In Windows 10, go to **Settings > System > Display** and toggle the **Night light** switch to turn on the feature.

Click the **Night light settings** link for additional settings. Use the slider to adjust the temperature of your screen. You can also put the feature on a schedule from sunset to sunrise or set it to go on and off at specific times.

In Windows 11, open **Settings > System > Display** and select **Night light**. Click the **Turn on now** button to activate the feature. You can then adjust the colour temperature by moving the slider on the Strength scale.

You can set up Night light so it automatically goes into effect at the right hours. Turn on the switch for **Schedule night light**. Here, you have two choices: Sunset to sunrise or Set hours. To set it for sunset to sunrise, you must have already enabled Location services in Windows.

If you prefer to set specific hours for Night light, click **Set hours**. Click the time under the **Turn on** line to set the start time. Then click the time under the **Turn off** line to set the time it stops. Night light will now automatically kick in when you need it and fade away when you don't.

Too Much Work? Try Blue Light Glasses Instead

Do you also suffer from eyestrain while staring at the computer? If you think it's too much work to set up these blue light filters on all your devices, blue light glasses can also help. We run through how they can help and which pairs might be best.

STEP 3 – DIETERY ADJUSTMENTS

Processed foods are known to be full artificial ingredients, e-numbers, hormones, and many other undesirable ingredients. Fast, busy and hectic schedules not to mention rising food costs impact on our likelihood of consuming a healthy, nutritional, naturally balanced diet. It would seem that more and more people are becoming aware of the long-term health benefits of embracing plant-based diets and becoming vegetarian or vegan. Recent statistics within the UK show that red meat sales have reduced by 20% within the last 18 months, which is actually good for the environment. Governments worldwide are now under pressure to raise awareness on the consumer but also to apply pressure to the manufactures on healthier options. Scandinavian dietary concepts such as sugar tax and scare branding are becoming widely adopted globally. Dietary changes are not only imperative for your health but from a government point of view or more cost effective in reducing NHS bills for long term terminally ill patients. There are also global initiatives in place now to drive down red meat consumption to help the environment as the methane gas produced by the animals in the farming industry are known to be tremendously harmful to our planet. More and more people are becoming, vegan, vegetarian and fully embracing the currently trending plant-based concept.

There exists some significant evidence to suggest dietary adjustments can help reduce or even cure your tinnitus symptoms. There are also many suggestions of various Vita biotic supplements that can be introduced to your diet to help. I'd like to remain consistent and not turn this into a science lesson, rather than bore you with another 100 pages of test results, experiments and case study, I'd like to educate you on what I know worked for me when I included this on my 3-year assault to collectively cure my tinnitus, so here goes.

Eliminate Caffeine

There is a high chance that you are not going to like this suggestion but seriously, if you are hell bent on easing your tinnitus-based suffering then this part of the plan is a deal breaker. Out of all of the things you eat and drink in a full 24 hours there are a few things to absolutely avoid but for now I want you to focus on just one - **Avoid caffeine**. If there is one prolific antagonistic ingredient to your daily dietary consumption then caffeine would be it. In the knowledge that tinnitus is usually triggered by erratic nerve impulses, without a scientific explanation how would you imagine caffeine impacts electro stimulated nerve signals in the brain? A widely acknowledged fact is that caffeine increases your heart rate, stimulates your brain and in most cases enhances your performance. Caffeine is mother nature's gift to staying wide awake. In most cases caffeine does a great deal of good but believe me, if you are a tinnitus sufferer caffeine in your public dietary enemy number 1.

In this book there exists no magic tricks or gimmick, you are aware that there is no magic pill to cure tinnitus but as far as tinnitus curing magic goes, caffeine reduction or when completely eliminated is the single most magical impactive piece of advice I can give you.

I think its relevant for me to tell you that before I suffered with tinnitus, I was a huge consumer of caffeine. The average daily recommended intake of caffeine for a (non-pregnant) adult is 400mg, that's approximately 4 cups of coffee or 10 cans of soda. It's safe to say my consumption was around double this amount, needless to say I had trouble sleeping, who knows maybe this is a factor in my initial tinnitus diagnoses. My morning cup of coffee was essential to the start of everyday, mid-morning would be another followed by a lunch time stimulation drink which included high doses of caffeine and taurine which was just enough to get me through until my 2pm coffee. Was I addicted to coffee, maybe? I prefer the words 'reliant upon' (another term for addicted - I know). Because I was so, ahem, reliant upon caffeine there were of course withdrawal symptoms as I begun the process of reducing my intake and progressed to completely eliminating from my diet. I suffered headaches, irritability, fatigue and extreme lethargy. In the first few weeks I noticed no change in my tinnitus as all, however after a few weeks I began to see huge reductions in my mid-day tinnitus observations. Its vital that I reiterate a multi-pronged assault was afoot to selfheal myself, therefore it would be unfair of me to solely attribute my cure to caffeine reduction. If that was the case this book would be about 5 lines in length and simply be entitled 'Stop consuming caffeine, your tinnitus will go'. Though it is by far the most tangible impactive magical suggestion I can offer you where you will hopefully see some rapid improvement.

Introduce more Zinc & Magnesium to your diet.

I introduced Zinc and Magnesium significantly into my diet and specifically in supplement form. Although I believe it contributed in my own healing don't just believe me, there are reams of research into the cognitive benefits of both zinc and magnesium, I have provided a little more detail below, also if you are not keen on supplements then I have also provided below two separate lists of food rich in Zinc & Magnesium foods which may wish to introduce into your diet instead of supplements.

Zinc

Zinc is a cofactor for enzymes that aid in many of the body's chemical reactions. Supplementing with 220 mg of daily zinc improved symptoms of tinnitus in a group of 40 tinnitus sufferers, according to the October 2002 "Auris Nasus Larynx." The Recommended Daily Allowance, RDA, for zinc is 11 mg for adult men and 8 mg for adult women, according to the Office of Dietary

Supplements. (Always consult your doctor before adding supplements)

Magnesium

Magnesium is an essential mineral that promotes healthy bone formation and helps nerves work properly. Research published in the July 2002 issue of "Otology & Neurotology" investigated the effect of magnesium on hearing loss and tinnitus 2. The researchers discovered that an intravenous-delivered magnesium compound improved symptoms of tinnitus in a significant number of research subjects. The current RDA for magnesium is 400 mg for men and 310 mg for women.

- Magnesium is an essential mineral that promotes healthy bone formation and helps nerves work properly.
- Research published in the July 2002 issue of "Otology & Neurotology" investigated the effect of magnesium on hearing loss and tinnitus 2.

17 Foods rich in Zinc

1. Oysters

2. Lamb

3. Pumpkin Seeds

5. Grass-Fed Beef

6. Chickpeas (Garbanzo Beans)

7. Lentils

8. Cocoa Powder

9. Cashews

10. Kefir or Yogurt

12. Mushrooms

13. Spinach

14. Avocado

15. Chicken

16. Almonds

17. Eggs

10 Foods Rich in Magnesium

1. Wheat bran

2. Amaranth

3. Spinach, cooked

4. Sunflower seeds, dried

5. Black beans

6. Mackerel

7. Cashews

8. Flaxseeds

9. Almonds/almond butter

10. Dark chocolate

STEP 4 – SLEEP Management

This may be a little on the obvious side but a lack of sleep can be a negative influence on a great many health issues, not least tinnitus. You must have heard or read about the importance of a good night's sleep, it's no secret that sleep is good for you. Almost every health agency globally openly promotes the benefits of a good night's sleep. On the off chance that you may not know about the necessity of sleeping lets just have a brief whistle stop tour.

Would your car run without a battery? Would your smart phone run without an overnight charge? Does a solar panel function without significant exposure to the sun? Of course not, none of these creations work without a little recharging or suitable replenishment. Our bodies, brains and vital organs work in a similar fashion. Although it is possible to function without sleep it is unlikely to benefit from any optimum performance, focus or drive. A couple of nights without sleep and you can quickly find yourself in a zombie like state and stumbling along in auto pilot. Not to mention a very short fuse and easily aggravated temper! I am undoubtably not alone in being a complete misery with no sleep. Why is this so important? What happens to us when we sleep that makes us feel so much better? When you fall into a state of sleep you transfer you mind from the conscious into the state of the unpredictable sub-conscience, this is where our dreams manifest. During this period of rest our autonomic nervous system takes control of our essential bodily functions and allows everything else to replenish and regenerate, especially this period of rest provides the opportunity for your brain to rejuvenate. Leading up to my tinnitus diagnoses collectively there was whole host of things that I was neglecting in my life and sleep was definitely one of them. Around this time, to say I was consistently getting 4 hours sleep was probably being quite generous, making sure I had 8 was very last on my agenda. Of course, it is rather easy for many people to simply put aside the time to bank 8 hours sleep a night, sadly that wasn't an option for me at the time even if I wanted too, I was a total insomniac or as its often described 'an overactive mind'. The problems here may appear obvious, if I'm drinking too much caffeine, my mind is more active, if my mind is more active, I cannot sleep, if I cannot sleep, I cannot replenish vital functions of my brain = tinnitus among other problems. I'd like you to take a leap of faith here and believe me that sleep is way up on the list of priorities in tinnitus reduction. Only you know if getting 8 hours is possible to you, achieving 8 hours was eventually achievable to me after investing in some lifestyle changes, in particular lifestyle changes listed in steps 1,2 & 3 above. A combination of caffeine reduction, less blue screen exposure (especially near bed-time), the introduction of some relaxation and breathing techniques just before sleep time and an overall conscious effort to regulate what we eat and drink will pay dividends. There is an abundance of pre-sleep videos on YouTube which include sounds of waves, rain and thunder or whatever sounds you find relaxing. The duplicate benefit here is the distraction noise and sounds being played can help to drown out the noise of the tinnitus. Equipped with a good set of Bluetooth sleep headphones and a carefully selected playlist you will be asleep in no time.

I fully appreciate this is much to take in, therefore it is time for us to quickly recap. So far in the steps taken to eliminate tinnitus you have read about the benefits of introducing focussed relaxation and breathing exercises, blue screen exposure and dietary changes. You are slowly building an arsenal of tools to make drastic life changing improvements but we are not done yet. This may be a good time in the book to stop and take stock of what you have learned and begin to commission a plan to introduce these changes into your lifestyle, even if it is one a week you will be making progress, assuming tinnitus is the equivalent to Rome, we know it wasn't built in a day and therefore you and me cannot be built in a day either, this journey is one careful step at a time. When you are ready let us continue on this journey and learn the last steps in your tinnitus recovery.

STEP 5 Introducing Exercise

The human body wasn't built to sit still. Sadly, these days most of us do allot more sitting still than we do anything else. Have you ever heard the term 'Use it or lose it'? I cannot emphasise how true this is. Imagine this; if you came to one of my seminars, 100 of you came, sat down, listened to the seminar but at the end decided to stay seated, in fact you stayed seated for the next 3 years, you did nothing but eat and drink, do you think at the end of those 3 years you would be able to simply get up and walk out? It is highly likely the muscles in your legs would have extremely degenerated, the bones, Cartlidge and tendons would have declined and potentially stiffened beyond repair. Essentially you would have lost use of your legs. The same applies to your brain and every other part of your body, you need to use it and use it all the time to promote optimum functionality. The human body is by far the greatest, most complex miracles ever created but that does not make it invincible, for this reason we must look after it, maintain it and utilise whatever functions are available to you. When we begin to neglect this is when the cracks quickly start to appear in many forms, in this instance we are highlighting tinnitus and how a lack of movement can be a definite negative impact.

For a very long period of time, I did very little, the very bare minimum of exercise. For me the negative impact of not doing exercise is almost immediate. After just a week I will notice weight gain, extreme lethargy, tiredness, lack of concentration, lack of confidence and as a result mild depression. These are just a few and the things that are visibly noticeable to me personally but imagine what is going on inside the body around the vital organs, imagine the visceral fat build up within the arteries. The symptoms of weight gain, sluggishness and so on are your bodies way of warning you that you need to start getting active.

In my experience the hardest part of exercise is getting started. For example, actually getting to the gym or actually getting out of the door to go for a run is by far the most difficult, once you're actually up and out doing the exercise that part isn't so bad. One of my all-time greatest feelings is that moment when you have completed an exercise session, you have showered and you are leaving the gym, in that moment I truly feel amazing! Working out stimulates oxygen to be circulated throughout your veins and vital organs, your brain is pumped full of endorphins, your mind is full of clarity and the stress you had before your work out has been disposed of, to me this is just amazing. Can you begin to imagine the positive impact of regular exercise is doing for our physical capability and our mental health? I don't think you can compare the benefits to any other known treatment available. I cannot imagine there is a GP anywhere in the world that would recommend not including exercise as a medicine to help the ailments he or she are confronted with. Unless of course there are some extreme cardiovascular restrictions.

Fortunately, I was able to re-introduce regular exercise into my life in collectively with the other steps discussed so far but this is not possible without a massive self-helping of self-discipline. I was able to begin a combination or cardio/weights along with swimming five times a week, generally Monday to Friday to aid my recovery. This is the one step that includes so many other benefits! In just 3 months Not only had my blood pressure reduced, cholesterol level's lowered dramatically, 36lbs lost in excess weight, increased mobility, vastly improved mental health, better sleeping patterns and of course notable tinnitus reduction. It is possible that this is the hardest of all the steps to introduce, especially if you were to commit like I did to five gyms sessions a week, essentially you are talking about 10 hours of training in a 168 week. Whatever you do as long as its more, even just a 20 minute walk each day will certainly quite literally be a step in the right direction. Exercise is a fine and effective medicine with a plethora of benefits. A general boost in your mood and the subsequent splurge of endorphins are a welcome distraction from the mind-numbing torture that tinnitus creates, half of the battle of course is distraction, once distracted we can begin heal. Let's take a closer look at the exercise types and dig into the science.

How Exercise Can Help

Exercise has a number of benefits for people with tinnitus. For one, it can help reduce stress and anxiety, which can aggravate tinnitus symptoms.

Exercise also releases endorphins, which have mood-boosting effects that can help offset the negative feelings that tinnitus can cause.

Additionally, exercise can help improve sleep patterns, and getting enough rest is important for managing tinnitus symptoms.

Finally, exercise can increase blood flow and oxygenation to the head and neck, which can reduce inflammation and help reduce tinnitus symptoms.

While more research is needed, it appears that exercise may be a potential treatment option for tinnitus. If you are affected by tinnitus, it is important to speak with your doctor to see if exercise might be a good option for you

The best exercises for tinnitus

The best exercises for tinnitus are exercises that help to improve blood circulation. Exercises that improve blood circulation can help to deliver more oxygen and nutrients to the inner ear, which may help to reduce the symptoms of tinnitus.

Additionally, exercises that help to improve muscle tone can also be beneficial, as they can help to reduce the likelihood of developing tension headaches, which can often be a common side effect of tinnitus.

Some of the best exercises for tinnitus include aerobic exercise, strength training, and yoga.

1. Aerobic exercise

One of the best exercises for tinnitus relief is aerobic exercise. Aerobic exercise gets your heart pumping and increases blood flow throughout your body, including to your ears. This increased blood flow can help to reduce the symptoms of tinnitus.

Swimming is also a great exercise for tinnitus sufferers because it does not put any additional pressure on the ears or sinuses. In addition, swimming can help to improve blood circulation and reduce stress levels. Just be sure to use earplugs if you are swimming in chlorinated water.

2. Strength Training

In addition to aerobic exercise, strength training is also a great way to help reduce tinnitus symptoms. Strength-training exercises help to increase blood flow and reduce inflammation throughout the body, both of which can help lessen tinnitus symptoms. Strength training can also help reduce stress levels, which can again make tinnitus more manageable.

There are many different ways to incorporate strength training into your routine. You can lift weights at the gym, do bodyweight exercises at home, or take a group fitness class. Start slow and gradually increase the intensity of your workouts as you get stronger. Aim for two or three strength-training sessions per week for best results.

However, keep in mind that if you overexert yourself or if you lift weights incorrectly, you can make things worse for yourself. In fact, weightlifting can even cause tinnitus if you push yourself too much.

3. Yoga

Yoga is another great exercise for tinnitus sufferers. Yoga helps to reduce stress levels and improve blood circulation. Yoga poses that are beneficial for tinnitus include Cow-Face Pose, Triangle Pose, Downward-facing Dog, and Cobra Pose.

Bhramari Pranayama, a yoga breathing technique, is also helpful for tinnitus. The technique involves exhaling slowly and deeply through the nose while making a humming noise. This helps to improve blood circulation and reduce stress levels.

4. Tai chi

Tai chi is a Chinese martial art that combines movement with meditation. Tai chi has been shown to be helpful in reducing stress levels and improving blood circulation. It is also an excellent way to focus on the present moment and clear your mind, which can help to lessen the symptoms of tinnitus.

5. Jaw stretches

Another effective exercise is to gently stretch your jaw muscles.

Jaw stretches are done by opening your mouth as wide as you can and then holding it for 30 seconds. There are also other jaw exercises you can try which you can find on .

6. Neck rolls

Another great way to help relieve tinnitus symptoms is to do some neck rolls. Start with your head tilted forwards, then slowly roll it backwards until you're looking up at the ceiling. Hold this position for a few seconds before slowly rolling your head back to the starting position. Repeat this 10-15 times, several times a day.

How to start an exercise program if you suffer with tinnitus

If you suffer from tinnitus, you may be worried that exercise will exacerbate your symptoms. However, there are a few simple steps you can take to make sure that your exercise program is safe and effective.

Firstly, it's important to consult with your doctor to get their approval before starting any new physical activity. Once you have the green light from your doctor, start slowly and gradually increase the intensity of your workouts. For example, you might begin by walking for 20 minutes a day and then add in some light weightlifting or swimming as you become more comfortable. It's also crucial to warm up before each workout and cool down afterwards. This will help to avoid sudden changes in blood pressure that could trigger tinnitus symptoms. Lastly, be sure to listen to your body and take breaks if you feel dizzy or lightheaded. By following these guidelines, you can safely enjoy the many benefits of exercise even if you have tinnitus.

How often should I exercise if I have tinnitus?

Aim for two or three strength-training sessions per week or 30 minutes of cardio each day. However, listen to your body and take breaks if you feel dizzy or lightheaded.

Why does my tinnitus get worse after exercise?

While exercise may help to lessen tinnitus symptoms for some people, for others it can actually make the condition worse. This is because when you exercise, your heart rate increases and blood pressure rises. If you have tinnitus, these changes in blood pressure can trigger or worsen the symptoms.

Should I lift weights if I have tinnitus?

While moderate aerobic exercise is generally considered safe for people with tinnitus, strenuous activities such as weightlifting can make symptoms worse. That's because lifting weights can cause a temporary increase in blood pressure, which can make tinnitus symptoms more pronounced. As a result, it is important to speak with a doctor before starting any new exercise regimen. In some cases, it may be necessary to modify your routine in order to find an activity that does not aggravate your condition.

What should I do if my symptoms worsen when I exercise?

If you experience any worsening of your tinnitus symptoms when you exercise, stop immediately and consult with your doctor. It's important to find an exercise routine that is safe and comfortable for you.

Can exercise cause tinnitus?

While the exact cause of tinnitus is not known, there are several potential risk factors that have been identified.

One of these is exposure to loud noise, which can damage the delicate hair cells in the inner ear. Exercise has also been suggested as a possible trigger for tinnitus, although the exact mechanism is not fully understood.

It is thought that strenuous exercise may lead to inflammation in the middle ear, which could in turn damage the hair cells and lead to tinnitus. While there is no definitive evidence that exercise causes tinnitus, it is important to be aware of this potential risk factor. If you experience ringing in your ears after exercising, it is advisable to see your doctor to rule out any other underlying causes.

Step 6 – Mind Control

The mind is an extraordinary tool laden with countless distractions which can either encourage positivity or negativity. Tinnitus is a scientifically proven entity, meaning in most cases something is physically happening inside the brain/inner ear to actually make this happen to you, in other words it's not a phantom existence. I have experienced tinnitus at its worst, met with many tinnitus patients and conducted tremendously in-depth research on the subject and extremely suffered. I wholeheartedly agree that something physical is happening however I do strongly believe the way we think can either positively or negatively on the impact on the severity of tinnitus. I would like to give you some examples of how positive mind-set can really help you.

During the first and second world war soldiers were provided with first aid field kits, within each kit was 2-3 doses of morphine to be injected into the blood stream in the event of a serious injury to reduce pain and provide relief. At one stage during the second world war Britain was weeks away from collapse at the hands of the German army. The British troops, especially those on the front-line were depleted of many crucial supplies including Morphine. There appeared to be no solution to this, however by trial, error and improvisation field medics began to discover a solution by administering an injured victim with sugared/clouded water (which looked like morphine) the sugar water had the exact same effect of pain relief as the morphine itself! How could this be? The answer is in the belief of the patient, they certainly were not told what they were being given they merely believed it. This method is widely known as the 'Placebo' effect. Since the second world war countless effective experiments have been conducted positively proving beyond reasonable doubt the effectiveness of 'The Placebo Effect'. Perhaps an even more concise example of this is a reversed version of this experiment. After the second world war thousands of soldiers were subject to the loss of limbs due to their injures, better known as amputees. When a person is subject to an amputation and almost unexplainable phenomenon is known to take place. For example, consider a victim of a land mine explosion who has lost his right leg below his knee, this kind of victim commonly reports to still suffer frequent and un-imaginable pain traceable to the area which no longer exists (the missing limb) In this example – the lower leg. Not only will the pain target this area of the body, the pain is frequently intolerable and no prescribed pain killers help to retract the pain. This could only mean that the pain is being self-orchestrated by the patient's brain, this is known as a phantom pain. So, if no pain killer can help, what is the solution? It isn't the re-introduction of the old limb, nor the fitting of an artificial one, the answer is bazaar but logical in many respects. After a few years of head scratching and many failed attempts to ease the phantom pain, doctors introduced ceiling mirrors to the bed bound patients. The idea behind this is to create an optical illusion of showing the patient that the limb is no longer attached to there body, the results of this are truly remarkable as the pain and suffering of amputee patients were almost instantly relieved of phantom pain. This is a tried and tested medical method used to the present day.

So how does injecting a patient sugar water or showing them a mirror impact on our tinnitus? It doesn't really, at least not directly but what it does achieve is heightened awareness surrounding the true power of our mind and its ability to play tricks on us. If a thing exists or not, it only matters if we believe it, therefore in theory if we adopt this theory, we can begin to indirectly apply

75

this to curing tinnitus. This is a key chapter in many respects as potentially this is the key to healing this and a great many other ailments. If you hold zero hope of anything in this book helping you, if you think you will simply obey the instructions but hold no belief the you may as well give up entirely as the battle is likely to already be lost. I want you to embrace the two examples I have just given you and apply them to your thought process, by doing this you are giving yourself every chance possible to make remarkable progress.

To summarise this step, we can conclude that the mind is an extremely powerful tool. It is my belief that tinnitus is part of the brain working against us and part of the recovery is journey is mind over matter and an ironclad belief that this can get better. I seriously believe that by positively charging and stimulating your thoughts you are giving yourself the best possible chance to make giant strides towards improvement. Henry Ford once said 'If you think you can do something or you think you can't, either way you are right'. Let those words sink for a moment before you move on.

Step 7 - Embracing Tinnitus

No matter how hard you try, tinnitus will never be defeated using brute force alone. Imagine tinnitus to be being a 500 lb solid muscle-clad wrestler that can breathe fire and crush its victims with a single blow, how do you defeat such a substantial enemy? Assuming you are not armed with nuclear missiles a machine gun or a tank you stand no chance to defeat this kind of enemy in a raw fist fight, the solution is trickery, you must outwit your opponent We must lure the beast into believing we are its friend and give it a big fat hug, must have heard of keeping your friends close and your enemies closer right?

Imagining your tinnitus is the beast that we describe above and imagine it is screaming at you for a fight, then the very worst thing you can do is scream right back at it, the more you fight it the stronger and more substantial the tinnitus will become. The taller you stand the taller your tinnitus will grow; you are ultimately feeding the beast. Instead consider this strange but effective concept as an option to temporarily provide you some much needed relief. Take a second to hear your tinnitus, but this time not only hear it, listen to it, listen hard for it, smile about it, if you are feeling really open minded get up and dance to the music of your tinnitus, imagine it is your very best friend! You must think I am crazy, go with it because I know it works. When you do this something weird and wonderful happens, the strength of the tinnitus begins to weaken and deteriorate and if you continue to listen, embrace and even dance for 10-15 minutes there is a very very good chance you won't hear it at all for a good few hours. The tinnitus beast will more than likely be more embarrassed than you and hide itself until you return to your normal vulnerable self. Please note that I have included this technique as a genuine quick fix to help you in desperate times, this among a few other techniques I will show you will arm you with good assortment of weapons to combat short term tin-attacks while we conjure up a long-term cure.

Step 8 – Cognitive Behaviour Therapy (CBT)

You may be a little surprised to see CBT listed as one of the steps in my cure strategy, when I first begun my tinnitus journey, I certainly was too. However, before you dismiss this and I explain in a little more detail how CBT actually works I want to explain how it worked for me. Before I began my CBT treatment, I was pessimistic to say the least, it just didn't seem feasible to me for this kind of treatment to work for me but low and behold it really did. In conjunction with the other steps, I felt a little like this was the icing on the cake for me. Much of the tinnitus battle is won by overcoming anxiety and one of the prominent by-products of CBT is anxiety management. CBT is exactly what it says on the tin – it's a form of therapy and being able to talk through the sufferance of my experiences and despair really felt like a big step forward and I left each session without the weight of the world on my shoulders. Below is a more in-depth explanation as to how it works, although be aware as always in this book an open mind is required to consider this treatment.

CBT uses techniques such as cognitive restructuring and relaxation to change the way patients think about and respond to tinnitus. Patients usually keep a diary and perform "homework" to help build their coping skills. Therapy is generally short-term — for example, weekly sessions for two to six months. CBT may not make the sound less loud, but it can make it significantly less bothersome and improve quality of life.

There is some low- to moderate-certainty evidence that CBT may reduce the negative impact that tinnitus can have on quality of life at the end of treatment, with few or no adverse effects (although further research on this is needed).

CBT is a form of talking therapy that aims to change the patient's emotional and/or behavioural response to their tinnitus. This review looked at studies of CBT for adults who had had tinnitus for at least three months. Participants in the control groups either received no intervention, audiological (hearing) care, tinnitus retraining therapy or another type of treatment. The review authors studied the effect of CBT on tinnitus-related quality of life, adverse effects, depression, anxiety, general quality of life and negatively biased interpretations of tinnitus.

When CBT was compared to no intervention there was low-certainty evidence that CBT may reduce the negative impact of tinnitus on quality of life at the end of treatment. It is not known whether this effect persists in the longer term (six or 12 months). There were few or no adverse effects (only one adverse effect was reported in one participant among seven studies). CBT may also slightly reduce depression (low-certainty evidence) and may reduce anxiety, although this finding is very uncertain. It is also uncertain whether CBT improves general quality of life or negatively biased interpretations of tinnitus.

Compared to audiological care, tinnitus retraining therapy and other types of treatment, there were findings that CBT probably reduces the negative impact of tinnitus on quality of life. The certainty of this evidence ranged from moderate to low. Where reported, there were few adverse effects and no significant differences between the groups. For depression, anxiety and general quality of life the results were more mixed and the evidence less certain. There is moderate-certainty evidence that CBT may reduce negatively biased interpretations of tinnitus compared to other types of treatment, but compared to audiological care and tinnitus retraining therapy the evidence is less certain.

My final thoughts on CBT are; Yes, it works, well it worked for me at least. Something to bear fully in mind is the costs involved and the availability of CBT therapists. CBT is expensive, it's cost per session varies anything from £65-£150 or for the American among you $80 - $180. Also, another issue is finding the availability of a CBT therapist, especially one who specialises in tinnitus.

Step 9 – Cannabis Derived Compound (CBD)

I appreciate the words don't fit the acronym, the first three letters "C", "B", "D" does not represent an abbreviated form of any three terms, so just so you know *CBD is technically not an acronym* at all

"CBD" is the short abbreviation for the specific cannabis-derived compound known as cannabidiol. Cannabidiol (CBD) is one of the many active compounds that are naturally produced in cannabis known as cannabinoids.
While there is still much to learn about these unique compounds, researchers have confirmed that cannabinoids are the source of the cannabis plant's various medicinal and recreational properties. Unlike some of the other cannabinoids, most notably Tetrahydrocannabinol (THC), CBD is a non-intoxicating compound, which means that it will not induce the mind-altering effects associated with "being high."
Essentially, CBD can deliver the natural, therapeutic properties of the cannabis plant, without the negative side effects of traditional cannabis use and importantly it is fully legal here in the UK, please check your own government guidelines surrounding the legality before use if you are outside the UK.

In keeping with the other steps outlined in this book and in the interests of consistent reading I'd like to again explore in a little more detail, open mindedness remains the key and a common theme running through this book like a stick of rock. Remember we are all different, what works for Peter may not work for Paul so please keep this in the forefront of your mind before adopting any of the steps included. Once again, I was perplexed at the possibility of including this particular step into my cure journey and perhaps more reluctant to begin CBD more than ay other step. First and foremost, I am anti-drugs, certainly illegal drugs and I include cannabis in that view point. Through school college, university and work-life I have always managed to avoid participating in the consumption of narcotics of all descriptions, when offered I would always walk away and make what I considered 'good choices' around drug use, so when the suggestion that CBD could be beneficial in helping with my tinnitus struggles, I almost immediately rejected the idea. It was only when I finally got my head around the fact that CBD wasn't narcotic in its nature. My research suggested it wasn't mood altering and it didn't lead to me getting 'high' it was quite the opposite. However, as I detail below there appeared to be enormous health benefits linked to taking CBD, benefits that couldn't be ignored. Once I had done my homework, established legality I flet like I had nothing to lose so I gave it a go starting with 3 drops under the tongue daily for two weeks. For the first three days I noticed no difference in anything, with other tinnitus reductions tactics well underway I didn't expect it to hugely impact positively on this in any case but I feel like it did. After a week or two of use I certainly felt an awe of tranquillity about myself, less anxious and I noticed some other positive bi-products so as improved mobility around my joints, less back pain after a workout. Undoubtably I was feeling the benefits of CBD. *One key thing to remember with CBD is you should always check the policy of acceptance from your employer before using it, although not illegal in the UK some employers frown upon its use and could potentially lead to you failing a work placed drug test, so do rigorously check your employer's stance on CBD before use, for example if you are operating machinery, driving or policing you will need to check the appropriacy.*

Once you nose-dive into the CBT rabbit hole you will discover many differences of opinion, you will also no doubt stumble across a few hundred stockists of this wonderous produce. My advice to you after carefully reading the research below is to find a reputable stockist and work with them to adopt the right strength for you. CBD comes in a variety of alternative strengths which should be taken as advised and proportionality to your height and build. As always before including this, read through the pros and cons in detail and always consult your GP.

How Does CBD Work?

While it was initially believed that cannabinoids were only found in cannabis, in the middle of the 20th century, researchers discovered that cannabinoids were produced in the body of most mammals as part of the Endocannabinoid system (ECS).

The ECS is comprised of millions of endocannabinoid receptors, which are classified into two groups: CB1 receptors and CB2 receptors.

The ECS is spread throughout the body in core health systems including the digestive system, central nervous system, cardiovascular system, and immune system. By utilizing the CB1 and CB2 receptors to relay neurological signals across the body, the ECS acts as a **biological communication system** that helps to moderate and maintain important functions throughout the body. CBD works by interacting with your bodies endocannabinoid system (ECS) this is a complex cell-signalling system identified in the early 1990s by researchers exploring THC, a well-known cannabinoid. Cannabinoids are compounds found in cannabis.

Experts are still trying to fully understand the ECS. But so far, we know it plays role in regulating a range of functions and processes, including:

- sleep
- mood
- appetite
- memory
- reproduction and fertility

The ECS exists and is active in your body even if you don't use cannabis. Read on to learn more about the ECS including how it works and interacts with cannabis. The ECS involves three core components: endocannabinoids, receptors, and enzymes.

Endocannabinoids also called endogenous cannabinoids, are molecules made by your body. They're similar to cannabinoids, but they're produced by your body. Experts have identified two key endocannabinoids so far:

- anandamide (AEA)
- 2-arachidonoylglyerol (2-AG)

These helps keep internal functions running smoothly. Your body produces them as needed, making it difficult to know what typical levels are for each.

Endocannabinoid receptors

These receptors are found throughout your body. Endocannabinoids bind to them in order to signal that the ECS needs to take action. There are two main endocannabinoid receptors:

- CB1 receptors, which are mostly found in the central nervous system

- CB2 receptors, which are mostly found in your peripheral nervous system, especially immune cells

- Endocannabinoids can bind to either receptor. The effects that result depend on where the receptor is located and which endocannabinoid it binds to.

- For example, endocannabinoids might target CB1 receptors in a spinal nerve to relieve **pain**. Others might bind to a CB2 receptor in your immune cells to signal that your body's experiencing inflammation, a common sign of autoimmune disorders.

Enzymes

Enzymes are responsible for breaking down endocannabinoids once they've carried out their function. There are two main enzymes responsible for this:

- fatty acid amide hydrolase, which breaks down AEA
- monoacylglycerol acid lipase, which typically breaks down 2-AG

What are its functions?

The ECS is complicated, and experts haven't yet determined exactly how it works or all of its potential functions. Research Trusted Source has linked the ECS to the following processes:

- appetite and digestion
- metabolism
- chronic pain
- inflammation and other immune system responses
- mood
- learning and memory
- motor control

- sleep
- cardiovascular system function
- muscle formation
- bone remodelling and growth
- liver function
- reproductive system function
- stress
- skin and nerve function

These functions all contribute to homeostasis, which refers to stability of your internal environment. For example, if an outside force, such as pain from an injury or a fever, throws off your body's homeostasis, your ECS kicks in to help your body return to its ideal operation. Today, experts believe that maintaining homeostasis if the primary role of the ECS.

How does THC interact with the ECS?

Tetrahydrocannabinol (THC) is one of the main cannabinoids found in cannabis. It's the compound that gets you "high." Once in your body, THC interacts with your ECS by binding to receptors, just like endocannabinoids. It's powerful partly because it can bind to both CB1 and CB2 receptors. This allows it to have a range of effects on your body and mind, some more desirable than others. For example, THC may help to reduce pain and stimulate your appetite. But it can also cause paranoia and anxiety in some cases. Experts are currently looking into ways to produce synthetic THC cannabinoids that interact with the ECS in only beneficial ways.

How does CBD interact with the ECS?

The other major cannabinoid found in cannabis is cannabidiol (CBD). Unlike THC, CBD doesn't make you "high" and typically doesn't cause any negative effects. Experts aren't completely sure how CBD interacts with the ECS. But they do know that it doesn't bind to CB1 or CB2 receptors the way THC does. Instead, many believe it works by preventing endocannabinoids from being broken down. This allows them to have more of an effect on your body. Others believe that CBD binds to a receptor that hasn't been discovered yet. While the details of how it works are still under debate, research suggests that CBD can help with pain, nausea, and other symptoms associated with multiple conditions.

Further research on tinnitus and CBD

Scientists have discovered two cannabinoid receptors in the brain, known as CB1 and CB2, that respond to the presence of cannabis and CBD. Emerging research shows that these receptors may play a role in balance and hearing. This has led some to wonder if taking CBD might help with hearing disorders, such as tinnitus. But there's not a lot of information to date.

A 2015 study using CBD to treat lab rats, for example, showed it didn't help, and in some instances even seemed to worsen tinnitus (in rats, at least). A 2020 literature review stated that human research is needed before any conclusions can be drawn.

However, there's some evidence that CBD might help with stress, which can be a problem for people with chronic tinnitus. For example, the results of a study published in the 2015 issue of *Neurotherapeutics* suggests CBD is effective in reducing anxiety behaviours related to disorders such as PTSD, SAD and OCD. Other studies have produced mixed results,

This lack of data also exists for side effects. Research suggest side effects may include; dry mouth, diarrhoea, reduced appetite, drowsiness and fatigue. CBD can also interact with other medications you're taking, such as blood thinners."

Research on CBD for tinnitus is mixed. It often appears contradictory, but there are many factors at play. The difficulty is that the way CBD affects the body is very complex. There are more than 100 phytocannabinoids, or types of cannabinoids, for example. The body also reacts differently to CBD, even for the same mixtures, with changes to drug formulation, route of taking it, and concentration of the CBD. Studies are ongoing to understand the many CBD receptor mechanics in different systems of the body. Tinnitus can also be caused by many different or unknown factors, making it difficult to pinpoint exact treatments. This can help explain why research will take time to give clear answers about CBD and tinnitus treatment.

What about endocannabinoid deficiency?

Some experts believe in a theory known as clinical endocannabinoid deficiency (CECD). This theory suggests that low endocannabinoid levels in your body or ECS dysfunction can contribute to the development of certain conditions. A 2016 article Trusted Source reviewing over 10 years of research on the subject suggests the theory could explain why some people develop migraine, fibromyalgia, and syndrome. None of these conditions have a clear underlying cause. They're also often resistant to treatment and sometimes occur alongside each other. If CECD does play any kind of role in these conditions, targeting the ECS or endocannabinoid production could be the missing key to treatment, but more research is needed.

STEP 1-9 Summary

You will be relieved to know we have now come to the end of my nine essential steps to tinnitus recovery. You are forgiven for maybe thinking this isn't going to be easy, the truth is it really won't be easy. I mentioned earlier in the book that some of the steps may not suit all readers but don't fret, just try and incorporate as many changes as possible and even if that change is just one small step, then you will still be making progress and heading in the right direction. In any case healing tinnitus is without doubt a marathon and not a sprint. Ultimately, I can only speak of my own experience, my own recovery and my own results however even though each step might seem like a lengthy read and allot to take in I thought it was crucial to back up my methods with the science, research and know-how.

CHAPTER 6

The 3 Step Cheat Sheet and Quick fixes

Now we have established the long-term remedies I'd like to arm you with some quick wins for those days when there is just no let-up from tinnitus. There are so many of these quick fixes listed online and in other books on this subject but I have discovered most of them to be mythical poppy-cock. Rest safe in the knowledge that I have once again acted in the capacity as the human Guinee-pig and tested most of the quick fixes, if not all and have whittled this list down to just three. They are as follows, but before trying any of them please remember these are not the longer-term solutions detailed earlies in the book, these are as the title of the chapter suggests - Quick fixes

Ear Trickery Flickery

This little trick is intended to buy you some time in moments of tinnitus desperation, maybe before an important meeting or when you are with friends are family. The effects will likely be positive but limited to approximately 30-40 minutes when you can once again repeat the process.

Here goes…. Hold both your hands over both ears in the cupping position, as if you are protecting them from a really loud sudden noise. With your hands cupped pressed against the ears, your fingers should naturally now rest on the skull just behind the ears. Now place your index finger on top of your middle (long finger) to gain some traction, then still while maintaining the cupping position on your ears allow the index finger to flick down on the skull behind the ear. Because you have the sound blocked out by cupping your ears you should hear a loud drumming base noise on the skull and within your ear. It shouldn't be painful and nor should you flick so hard that it should hurt in any way, but you should hear it quite loudly. Repeat this process approximately 30-40 times in about a 1-minute session. Immediately after doing so, you should then observe immediate tinnitus relief, albeit very temporary it is a minor escape mechanism, but as I have said that is all it is and nothing more. I would only advise using this technique a maximum of 3 times in any 24-hour period to avoid causing any damage or irritation to this area.

In summary;

> 1. Place the palms of your hands over your ears so your fingers wrap around the back of your head.

2. Set your middle fingers on the top of your neck right at the base of your skull.
3. Put your index fingers on top of your middle fingers and apply pressure.
4. Now snap them on the back of your head over and over like you're drumming

Menthol Vapour Rub

This handy little trick doesn't always work but it is something to be aware of and perhaps harmlessly experiment with. Tinnitus is linked quite significantly to the central nervous system and therefore is susceptible to stimulants that cause-and-effect changes to this. You are probably aware that the Ear nose and throat are also linked, therefore some medicines used to treat their areas i.e., nasal sprays and lozenges have surprisingly been known to effect tinnitus in subtle ways. One of the most commonly widely used products is over the counter menthol-rub. Without actually applying any menthol rub directly into the ear or the nose, try applying a little directly onto your top lip, just below the nose, also apply a very small amount on the outer edges of the ear. The idea of this will seem a little strange but often this can have a fast-acting positive impact on reducing the severity of tinnitus for a short while. Referring to my own experience I can vouch for the fact that my tinnitus would often worsen during times of illness, usually when having a cold or sinus infection. Without providing you with a scientific explanation as to why this helps elevate the severity, I can tell you that it did help me/ This technique may or may not help you but if anything, I do appreciate that tinnitus causes people to become exceptionally desperate for answers, tinnitus is a subject for which there are few answers from most, therefore every little helps right?

Headphones, fans and background buzzing

Long term tinnitus sufferers by default often come up with their own helpful techniques to ease the suffering. Having mentioned silence as a common enemy a few times in this book I want to share with you a few day-to-day items I have used to help me and others. As the night time silence would loom and day turned to dusk I would prep my bedtime procedure to eliminate silence. I would always have a few headphone choices by my bedside. This would include one set which has Bluetooth speakers built into a cushioned headband, may have just been one of the best gadgets I ever purchased. I would often listen to audio-books, sounds of nature, waves, dolphins and the like to help me drift of the sleep without the distraction. There are machines that you can purchase which sit by your bed and play these kinds of sounds including white noise, however I didn't find these as effective as actually applying headphones (comfortable ones). The trick is to distract and divert the noise enough to actually get yourself to sleep, once you are asleep you are unable to hear your tinnitus, I know I certainly couldn't and I am yet to meet a tinnitus patient who could hear his or her tinnitus during a period of sleep.

Another great ally in any quest to get to sleep is the introduction of a bedtime fan. I found the constant whirring noise and the welcome fresh breeze to be of great distraction and comfort in my tinnitus experience. During my worst episodes of tinnitus, I can remember struggling to even think about getting to sleep without my fan on. I guess it is partly what you get used too, for me headphones and a fan were a total godsend and a welcome addition to my bedtime preparation.

CHAPTER 7

Miscellaneous Cures

I thought long and hard about including this chapter of the book, however I feel like you would be getting a bit of a dis-service from me if I didn't. I want to include some information around some of the other available cures out there and available. The reason they have been listed in as 'miscellaneous' is that I haven't tried them and not in the best position to provide you with the best advice although if you do your own research, you will discover there are plenty of people who have tried some of the 'alleged cures' which I will write about next, some successfully, some not so successful. I'd like to think that overall, this book not only has given you my sympathy, advice, understanding and knowledge but also provided you with a broad understanding of the global solutions to this problem. Ideally, I would like you to come away from this with a wide spectrum of understanding which will allow you to make all the right choices for you.

Tinnitus Surgery

The first cure listed in this section is a bit of a biggie! It's a tinnitus operation. I would personally never consider such a thing as from my own understanding once surgeons start interfering with complexities of the inner ear, brain and inner skull then as far as I am concerned it's a total can of worms and presents great risk. That said my research suggests this is an operation that has been done successfully on many occasions but has also had some failures and in some unsuccessful operations has caused some pretty horrendous outcomes. Although the surgery option exists for each extreme generic tinnitus suffers the surgery option is mainly used for suffers with pulsatile tinnitus, this is basically all of the usual symptoms of tinnitus but the sufferer will be able to actually here there-own pulse. I was never a long term-sufferer of pulsatile tinnitus but I did actually experience it for a short time, for around a day or two. Let me tell you pulsatile tinnitus is about as annoying as it gets and I have complete and utter sympathy for those who suffer this type of tinnitus. Let's talk a bit about what the surgery does and how it works.

In these procedures, the surgeon cuts into the blood vessel and removes the relevant obstruction. If the irregular blood vessel was indeed the cause of the offending noise, the symptoms should soon cease completely.

There are also less invasive procedures for the treatment of pulsatile Tinnitus. Some cases are caused by venous sinus stenosis, which affects the veins in the brain. A treatment involving stenting the narrowed veins is now in a promising clinical trial and is worth keeping an eye on.

If successful, the treatment will alleviate the obstruction to blood flow in the area and drastically reduce tinnitus. A patient undergoing this procedure can expect to be hospitalized for only 1-2 days.

In some cases, the noise can be caused by a cyst or tumour pinching on the auditory nerve. When Tinnitus appears under these circumstances, there is a physically removable source. Not surprisingly, these instances are most conducive to successful surgery.

One of the most commonly performed tinnitus-related surgeries involves the removal of acoustic tumours (vestibular schwannoma). These are non-cancerous tumours that can develop on the main nerve connecting the brain to the inner ear. Though this is one of the most straightforward surgeries related to Tinnitus, it only improves the malady in 40% of the cases.

Another promising procedure for tinnitus caused by tumours is the use of surgical cochlear nerve decompression. In this type of surgery, a portion of the bone or disk material near the nerve root is removed to provide more space. Though controversial, one study shows that the procedure has a 52% success rate in reducing long-term symptoms in relevant cases.

Hearing-Aid for tinnitus

You suffer with ringing in your ears but not necessarily suffering with hearing loss or deafness? How on earth can hearing aids help? Again, this is another treatment which seems successful for many but not all. I have tried this for a very short period, once again not for any length of time for me to be able to comment either way. I can tell you though hearing aids are a bit of surreal experience. If you are yet to try it this is how I would describe it. It kind of feels like you have been transported into a computer game, radio or television. Everything all of a sudden sound a bit 'synthetic' and 'tinny'. The theory behind this is that the aid masks the tinnitus with synthetic background sound. This definitely wasn't for me for a couple of reasons, firstly because the choice between tinnitus and constant synthetic background sounds would lead me to choose tinnitus every time and being a relatively young man, it felt a little premature for me to be wearing hearing aids - this is purely from a superficial point of view and

perhaps a little vein of me but I am just being honest.
The hearing aid I was given really wasn't subtle and for
quite a few reasons this really wasn't a medium- or
longer-term option for me. Let's look at the finer details
of how this can potentially help you though.

**How Much Tinnitus Relief Can Hearing Aids
Provide?**

There is no exact number-answer to this question. The
best data available from my own online research where it
suggests from 175 audiologists, 48 hearing instrument
specialists and 7 professionals surveyed who specialise
in hearing loss and audiology in the United States and
Canada showed the following findings from the
introduction of hearing aids/

- 16.6% experienced minor relief
- 21.4% experienced moderate relief
- 22.1% experienced major relief
- 1.7% experienced a worsening of their
  Tinnitus
- 39% found no relief

How Do Hearing Aids Provide Tinnitus Relief?

Hearing aids provide Tinnitus relief by helping you hear
frequencies that you couldn't hear before. When your
brain receives auditory signals from your ears that it
didn't receive before, it shuts off the Tinnitus sound it

invented to compensate for your hearing loss in the first place.

Hearing aids do this by;

Enhancing environmental noise – Allow you to hear environmental sounds that you couldn't hear before. The supply of new auditory inputs will make your brain focus less on the Tinnitus, sometimes even helping it completely ignore the ringing.

By Stimulating Auditory Pathways – Hearing aids make your auditory pathways healthy again. Promotion of general auditory health betters your chance of experiencing Tinnitus relief or even resolution.

By Reducing Stress and Anxiety – When the ringing is all that you can hear and think about, your body and mind is subject to a lot of stress and anxiety. **Stress makes Tinnitus worse.** Hearing aids can help you normally hear people talk again. You can have conversations and focus on a social life. This can in turn allow you to reduce stress and anxiety and give your Tinnitus a chance to take a back seat or resolve itself.

How to Choose Hearing Aids That Can Help You with Tinnitus?
If you think hearing aids can help you find Tinnitus relief after reading all the information above, here's how you should go about choosing the best hearing aids to help you with your Tinnitus.

Affording it

Hearing aids are expensive. In the UK, they can cost anywhere between £500 to £4000 $700-$4500. Please remember that hearing aids have to be customized to suit your individual hearing profile. Buying online hearing aids with no personalized configuration can result in over-amplification or under-amplification that can make your hearing and Tinnitus much worse.
Your journey to buy hearing aids for Tinnitus MUST begin at an audiologist's office, in the UK the aid is normally customised and provided for by the NHS unless you choose the private route and a more expensive/advanced hearing aid

Two Hearing Aids are Better than One

You ideally want hearing aids that are bilateral or go on both ears. Using hearing aids on only just one ear can affect auditory symmetry that can make your Tinnitus or hearing loss worse in the long run.

Masking Feature

Many hearing aids designed to provide Tinnitus relief come with a masking feature. This is when the hearing aid can provide both amplification and also a soothing white noise like sound (waves, rain, fire etc) to help you focus less on your ringing.

While masking is useful to distract yourself from Tinnitus, you must know that it only provides a temporary relief. But, if the masking frequency can exactly match your Tinnitus frequency, you can essentially not hear the ringing anymore. Learn more about how and if Tinnitus masking works here. Hearing aids with masking can however drive up the cost of hearing aids quite a bit.

An Open-Fit

Ideally, you want an open-fit pair of hearing aids. These deliver amplified sounds that are delivered by a tube-like speaker directly into the ear canal. Such hearing aids can prevent what is called an occlusion or resonance effect. In other words, amplified sounds will not sound like you are sticking your head into a barrel.

Alternative Medicine & Therapies for tinnitus

This is my final offering in this book and honestly this is a subject worthy of its own book. I am a big fan of alternative medicine and healing but not necessarily for tinnitus. I have had my fair share of rai-ki, chi-gong and yoga classes. I can see how all of these methods can be of benefit. One of the most common alternatives used globally is acupuncture. I love acupuncture and have used it to help heal a variety of problems, I have found it particularly beneficial for sciatica and stress. When I asked my acupuncture therapist if he could help me cure my tinnitus (Bearing in mind I was paying £70-$85 per hour) advised me it absolutely doesn't help. I am certain though I could have visited a thousand other acupuncturists who would have taken my money and told me it would and maybe they are right as there is a plethora of research to suggest it does. Let's look at it more closely.

How does it work?

Strictly speaking Acupuncture is regarded as a traditional Chinese medicine rather than an alternative medicine. It works under the basis that your health depends on the flow of qi (energy) in your body. This energy travels along invisible pathways, known as meridians. These are found throughout your body.

Qi is believed to help keep your body in balance and promote its natural ability to heal itself. A blocked or disrupted flow of qi can negatively impact physical and emotional well-being.

During an acupuncture session, very thin needles are inserted into your skin to stimulate certain points, based on the symptoms you're addressing. This stimulation, according to TCM, helps to clear blockages along your meridians, restoring the flow of qi through your body.

What does the research say?

A number of studies have looked at acupuncture as a treatment for tinnitus. Results are mixed, but many recent studies suggest acupuncture may decrease the intensity of tinnitus, boosting quality of life. Results of a 2018 study in the United States which reviewed 88 adults with tinnitus suggest that acupuncture could help make tinnitus sounds quieter and less severe. A 2016 study similarly found that acupuncture likely helps with tinnitus. However, the authors noted that some of the studies they looked at were flawed and potentially biased. In addition, these studies often used different points, so it's hard to compare their results. Still, there's no evidence that acupuncture will make tinnitus worse, so it may be worth trying if you're interested.

Is it safe to try?

When performed by a trained and experienced acupuncturist, acupuncture is fairly safe, according to the National Centre for Complementary and Integrative Health Trusted Source.

But if acupuncture isn't performed correctly or needles aren't sterile, you may be at risk for serious side effects. Licensed acupuncturists in the United States must use disposable needles, so receiving acupuncture from a licensed professional should minimize your risk of complications. Find a licensed practitioner in your own state through your board of health.

Some people do experience mild side effects after an acupuncture, session, including:

- nausea
- dizziness
- pain or tenderness around the involved areas

It's also best to avoid acupuncture if you:

- are pregnant, as some points can induce labour
- have a pacemaker, which could be affected by the mild electric pulse that's sometimes used with acupuncture needles
- take blood thinners or have a bleeding disorder

How can I try acupuncture?

If you've decided to give acupuncture a try, it's essential to choose a qualified acupuncturist. The National Certification Commission for Acupuncture and Oriental Medicine (NCCAOM) offers licensing programs and examinations, but specific licensing requirements vary by state.

When looking for an acupuncturist, keep in mind that a licensed acupuncturist is not the same as a certified acupuncturist. Doctors, dentists, and other medical professionals may have certification in acupuncture and a few hundred hours of training, but they may have less experience working with patients.

Licensed acupuncturists, on the other hand, typically have a few thousand hours of training and must treat many of people under supervision before being licensed.

You can also ask your primary care physician for a referral or search the NCCAOM acupuncturist registry. Once you've found a provider, you can call your state licensing board to make sure they're licensed to practice in your state.

Things you might ask before making an appointment include:

- how long the acupuncturist has been working with clients
- whether they've treated sinus issues with acupuncture before
- how long treatment will take
- whether they accept insurance or offer a sliding-scale payment system

If you're worried about pain or discomfort, let them know. They may be able to address your concerns and help you feel more comfortable before your first session.

Even if the acupuncturist you choose accepts insurance, not all insurance providers cover acupuncture, so it's a good idea to call your provider to find out if they'll cover acupuncture treatments — and if so, how many.

CHAPTER 8 – THE HOME STRAIGHT

I offer you my most sincere congratulations for coming to the end of this book. I genuinely hope as a fellow (former) sufferer that I have been able to help you in some way. I said at the beginning you have my deepest sympathy for having to deal with tinnitus, perhaps once you have finished this book you might consider passing on to those who are part of your life who do not suffer in the hope that they too will sympathise is some way. If this book hasn't been able to help you with one of the methods, I have suggested then I do hope at the very least you have broadened your knowledge of tinnitus which will hopefully lead you to the solution and outcome you are looking for. As part of my genuine interest in your experiences, my ongoing research and curiosity please feel to email me at info@tinnitushope.com. I am deeply interested in your experiences and feedback on this book and will try my best to respond to you, I do get a tremendous number of emails so please bear with me I will get back to you eventually.

Lastly, I would like to wish you the very best of luck in you making a full tinnitus recovery, remember you are not alone and the support is out there if you look for it. As promised, I will leave you with the quick reference list for the steps to recover below.

1) Breathing Focus

2) Electronic device/blue screen reduction

3) Dietary Changes

4) Manage your sleep

5) Introduce regular exercise

6) Be a master of your own thoughts

7) Embrace tinnitus

8) Cognitive Behaviour Therapy (CBT)

9) Cannabis Oil (CBD)

I sincerely hope you have enjoyed reading this book and I truly hope it has helped you. My thoughts, prayers and good will remain with you - Jake Sutton

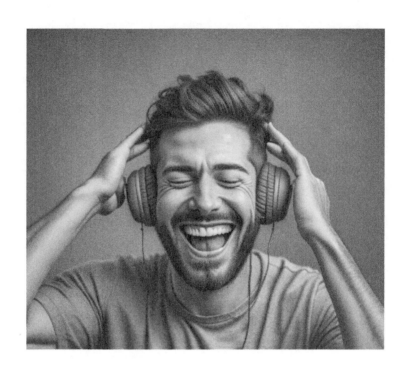

Printed in Great Britain
by Amazon

25046060R00066